Where Reincarnation
and Biology Intersect

Where Reincarnation and Biology Intersect

Ian Stevenson, M.D.

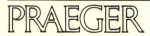

Westport, Connecticut
London

Library of Congress Cataloging-in-Publication Data

Stevenson, Ian.
    Where reincarnation and biology intersect / Ian Stevenson.
      p.   cm.
    Includes bibliographical references and index.
    ISBN 0–275–95188–X (alk. paper). — ISBN 0–275–95189-8 (pb. : alk.
paper)
    1. Reincarnation.   2. Birthmarks.   3. Abnormalities, Human—
Aetiology.   I. Title.
BL515.S754   1997
133.9'01'3—dc20   95–34442

British Library Cataloguing in Publication Data is available.

Library of Congress Catalog Card Number: 95–34442
ISBN: 0–275–95188–X
      0–275–95189–8 (pbk)

First published in 1997

Praeger Publishers, 88 Post Road West, Westport, CT 06881
An imprint of Greenwood Publishing Group, Inc.

Printed in the United States of America

The paper used in this book complies with the
Permanent Paper Standard issued by the National
Information Standards Organization (Z39.48–1984).

10 9 8 7 6 5

For Dr. Thomas Hunter
    a great Dean,
    profoundly skeptical of this research,
    equally defensive of the right to conduct it

Contents

Illustrations

Preface

This book introduces and condenses a much longer one entitled *Reincarnation and Biology: A Contribution to the Etiology of Birthmarks and Birth Defects*. That work is a medical monograph with extensive documentation, references, numerous tables, and many footnotes. This book has none of these. I have written it to satisfy the needs of readers who wish to understand the essential content of the larger work without troubling themselves over details. Let it be read as a series of abstracts. A good abstract in a scientific journal excites the reader's interest and entices him or her to read the complete article it summarizes. If this book persuades readers to study its parent monograph, I shall have succeeded in what I intended it to do.

A reader can only fairly judge the kinds of cases these books describe by close attention to their many details; and I do not believe anyone should express an opinion about my conclusions without having met this condition. This may seem censorious; but I say it to emphasize that the present work does not fully deploy the evidence in the cases. What readers have here are brutally shortened summaries. As I have omitted many strengths, so I have left out many weaknesses. The larger work presents in detail descriptions of flaws and discrepancies in the testimony of informants and defects in the investigations of the cases. Here all roughness has been smoothed out, not for deception but solely for brevity. (The few exceptions where I have mentioned weaknesses in the cases touch on details that seem to me especially important.) I often give the subject's birth date (or the year of birth), but otherwise I rarely mention dates except when one is relevant to a particular feature of the case, such as when a birthmark was examined or a photograph taken.

Because this book was printed after the monograph, I was able to add to it a few items of additional information about one case that I received too late for inclusion in the monograph. (This is the case of Ma Myint Myint Zaw in Chapter 12.) I have also clarified a discrepancy that remains without comment in the monograph. Otherwise, apart from the drastic abbreviation, the contents of this book correspond to those of the monograph.

Readers who wish to follow my advice and study details of a case in the monograph can easily find the longer case report, because I have given the chapters of this synopsis the same titles as those of the monograph, and within a chapter the case reports have the same order they have in the larger work. (In a few instances I have found it appropriate to describe a case in this book in a chapter different from the one of the monograph with the same chapter title in which the detailed report of the case appears; I have drawn attention to such exceptions where they occur.) In addition, Appendix D of the monograph lists alphabetically all the subjects in it and in this book and gives the chapters in which they are reported; the Index of Cases in the monograph gives the page numbers for the detailed case reports and other mentions of cases.

Colleagues have sometimes expressed curiosity and even dismay over the massive size of the larger work. I could have made it shorter, but instead it grew longer. I made it so because I am convinced that when several or many cases have similar features their numbers support the authenticity of the individual members of the group. For example, one case with a subject having birthmarks on the ear said to correspond to holes pierced for earrings deserves little attention; it may be an unimportant coincidence. After finding one such case, however, I continued to learn about and investigate others. Now readers of my larger work can study reports of nine such cases from four different cultures. For cases with some other features I have many more than nine examples. The inclusion of multiple examples accounts for most of the large size of the monograph. It contains reports—most of them detailed—of 225 cases, whereas this book provides summaries of only 112 cases. Of these cases, I have myself examined all but 8 of the subjects. In 3 cases, the subject had died before I investigated the case. In 5 other cases, I have used information furnished to me by associates and assistants.

A second, equally important, reason for the size of the larger work derives from the medical documentation that I have been able to furnish for a little more than one fifth of all the cases it describes. Postmortem reports and other medical documents should be detailed if they are to be of any value; and their interpretation may take as many lines as their citation.

For the more important chapters having case reports in this book I have included one or more photographs illustrating the birthmarks and birth defects. I have also indicated photographs and (sometimes sketches) that are published in the monograph by inserting an asterisk (*) after a reference in this book to the abnormality in question.

I said earlier that this book contains no references. I am trying the experiment of writing a book of science without them. Here again, however, readers can readily find the references for statements and quotations in this book by consulting the corresponding chapter of the monograph and by using its Indexes. Also, at the end of this book I give a list of books and papers in which some of my colleagues and I have published detailed case reports.

A Note on Real Names and Pseudonyms

The names used in these studies are a mix of real names and pseudonyms. I have used pseudonyms almost exclusively in certain areas (Western Europe and the Americas, for example) and, of course, when informants asked me to do so or when I thought that the person should be shielded from possible intrusions on his or her privacy.

For the same reasons, the names of towns or villages figuring in a case are not necessarily the names of the actual locations. However, when geographical factors, such as distances between communities, bear on the understanding or interpretation of a case, I have given them as precisely as I can.

This work abridges a medical monograph, although it touches on several branches of knowledge outside medicine. I did not have a professional medical relationship with any of the subjects of the cases; yet most of them knew that I am a physician, and this knowledge probably increased their willingness to allow medical aspects of their cases to be studied and themselves to be photographed. Accordingly, I believe that their privacy should be respected.

Persons wishing additional details about a case should write to me and provide sufficient information about their research strategies and purposes to warrant my providing such details.

Acknowledgments

In the larger work of which this book is a synopsis, I acknowledged numerous debts for assistance from many persons and institutions. I had thought that my thanks expressed there might suffice for this shorter volume; but they do not. As I wrote this book I had many pleasant memories of the generous and efficient assistance I received, from four persons in particular, during sometimes arduous field trips. In this short work when, for the sake of brevity, I say *we,* I nearly always mean to refer to one of these four. They are: the late Reşat Bayer (Turkey), the late U Win Maung (Burma, now Myanmar), Dr. Satwant Pasricha (India), and Godwin Samararatne (Sri Lanka).

I have also received much assistance during field trips from many other persons, including Dr. Chien Siriyanand, Nasib Sirorasa, the late Francis Story, the late Tem Suvikrom, and the late Dr. Kloom Vajropala (Thailand); Majd Mu'akkasah Dean (Lebanon); Tissa Jayawardene (Sri Lanka); the late U Tin Tut (later the Ven. U Dhammadara), U Nu, the late Daw Hnin Aye, Sujata Soni, the late Dr. R. L. Soni, and Maung Aye Kyaw (Burma); the late Patrick Onyekelu and Nicholas Ibekwe (Nigeria); Dr. Jamuna Prasad, Dr. L. P. Mehrotra, the late K. S. Yadav, Chandra Prakash, and K. S. Rawat (India).

Several other assistants, associates, and colleagues have conducted interviews or otherwise provided information that I have included in the case reports, and for this I thank: Dr. Stuart Edelstein (Nigeria and Senegal); Dr. David Barker and Dr. Antonia Mills (British Columbia); Issam Abul-Hisn, Dr. Emily Williams Cook, and Dr. Sami Makarem (Lebanon); Champe Ransom, Roxanne Turner, and Betty Hulbert (Alaska); Tosio Kasahara (Japan); Dr. Nicholas McClean-Rice, Parmeshwar Dayal, the late Professor P. Pal, Dr. Kirti Rawat, G.S. Gaur, Dr. Poonam Mittal, and Manjula Kamal (India); Ertan Kura, Dr. Can Polat, and Dr. Jürgen Keil (Turkey); Hernani Guimarães Andrade and Waldomiro Lorenz (Brazil); Dr. Erlendur Haraldsson, Dr. Nandadasa Kodagoda, and Hector Samararatne (Sri Lanka).

Financial support for the research reported in this work came mainly from the donations and bequest to the University of Virginia of the late Chester Carlson to whom I remain forever grateful. I have also received some additional assistance from the Fetzer Foundation, the James S. McDonnell Foundation, the Bernstein Brothers Parapsychology and Health Foundation, the Parapsychology Foundation, the Nagamasa Azuma Fund, and several anonymous donors.

Despite the abundance of the support just mentioned, publication of the large monograph faltered, until a generous donation from Ralph E. Fash of the Fash Foundation moved it forward again. To him I cannot sufficiently express my gratitude.

Dolly Ware played an important part in helping the project toward completion, and if I should not say here how she did this I can nevertheless give her my thanks.

These acknowledgments would remain shamefully incomplete without my thanks to the subjects of the cases here reported and to the other informants for them. I never counted them, but they number several thousand at least. For their patience in answering all my questions—which they may often have thought interminable—and for much gracious hospitality I am deeply thankful.

I am indebted to the Master and Fellows of Darwin College, Cambridge, whose hospitality enabled me to write the draft of this book.

With two exceptions all the photographs were taken by me or my associates, or at my request. The exceptions are Figure 1, reproduced by kind permission of *The Lancet,* and Figure 32, reproduced courtesy of Jagdish Chandra.

Dr. Emily Cook has given the text the kind of thorough review that has made her for years my most valued colleague. I am also grateful to Dr. Patrick Fowler, Dawn Hunt, and Dr. Antonia Mills for their careful readings of the book and the valuable comments that they gave me for its improvement.

To Patricia Estes I again owe heartfelt thanks for her careful attention to many details through many revisions. James Matlock contributed greatly by making the Index. Dawn Hunt gave additional assistance in the preparation of the Index. Melody Counts assisted in making the statements in this abridgment accord with those in the large monograph.

I once more thank my wife, Margaret, for her unselfish encouragement during the writing of this synopsis.

I dedicate this book to Dr. Thomas Hunter, former Dean of the School of Medicine at the University of Virginia. My debt to him is far greater than my poor words can adequately express.

1

INTRODUCTION

Children who claim to remember a previous life have been found in most countries where they have been sought. Reports of such children occur frequently in countries and cultures in which the belief in reincarnation is strong: the Hindu and Buddhist countries of South Asia, the Shiite peoples of Lebanon and Turkey, the tribes of West Africa, and the tribes of northwestern North America. We also have many (but fewer) reports of cases from Europe, North America, and elsewhere. I have published some 70 detailed reports of such cases, and, in recent years, several colleagues have published between them reports of another 15 cases.

I have deliberately referred to *reported* cases in the various countries and cultures that I mentioned. I use this word to emphasize that we have little information about the real incidence of the cases. In the 1970s a systematic survey of cases in a district of northern India showed that about one person in 500 claimed to remember a previous life. There are grounds for thinking that the incidence of cases may be higher in Lebanon and among the tribes of northwestern North America, but we have no figures from surveys that might confirm this opinion.

The cases are certainly found more easily in the non-Western countries and cultures that I mentioned earlier. Their strong belief in reincarnation allows a child who wishes to speak about a previous life to do so without being disbelieved or rebuked as such a child may be in the West. I believe, however, that the reasons for finding cases more readily in some non-Western cultures than in Western ones are deeper than the simple matter of permission for a child to speak about a previous life. This work is not the proper place to consider such an important topic. I would say, however, to Western readers: Do not make the mistake of thinking that because a phenomenon occurs more often in India than in your neighborhood it is no concern of yours. I say this for two reasons. First, a case may have occurred in your neighborhood without you (or I) knowing about it. Second, and more important, if reincarnation should prove to be the best interpretation of these cases, wherever they occur, this would have important implications for all of us.

1

In most of these cases the evidence consists mainly of statements from informants, often recorded months or even years after the case has developed. Such cases suffer from the serious defect that the accuracy of the informants' memories may have diminished with the passage of time; even worse, the two families concerned in a case may have mingled their memories and given the child more credit for accuracy in its statements than it deserves. It is possible to exaggerate these sources of weakness, but it is foolish to ignore them. In a small number of cases, however, we—by which I mean my colleagues and myself—have been able to reach the scene of a case within weeks of its development. In a still smaller number—only about 1% of the 2600 cases in our collection—someone, usually a member of our team, has made a written record of what the child has stated about the previous life before anyone verified these statements, and we have then verified them ourselves.

During my first visit to Sri Lanka in 1961 I investigated the case of Wijeratne (*), who had a severe birth defect said to derive from a previous life. (An asterisk after the name of a subject means that the monograph has a relevant figure or figures.) A few months later—on the other side of the world, in Alaska— I studied the cases of Charles Porter (*) and Henry Elkin (*). They were Tlingits who had birthmarks respectively related to a fatal stabbing with a spear and a gunshot wound. Despite this early introduction to the occurrence of birth defects and birthmarks in these cases, it took several years before I fully appreciated the importance of this type of case. Once I had this insight, I conceived the plan of collecting the reports of many such cases into a single large work.

The cases having birthmarks and birth defects are important for three reasons. First, the birthmarks and birth defects provide an objective type of evidence well above that which depends on the fallible memories of informants. We have photographs (and occasionally sketches) which show the birthmarks and birth defects. And for many of the cases, we have a medical document, usually a postmortem report, that gives us a written confirmation of the correspondence between the birthmark (or birth defect) and the wound on the deceased person whose life the child, when it can speak, will usually claim to remember. As I shall explain later, despite the obvious difficulties that the concept of reincarnation poses for Western thought in general and modern science in particular, the birthmarks and birth defects in these cases do not lend themselves easily to explanations other than reincarnation.

Second, the birthmarks and birth defects derive importance from the evidence they provide that a deceased personality—having survived death—may influence the form of a later-born baby. I am well aware of the seriousness—as well as the importance—of such a claim and can only say that I have been led to it by the evidence of the cases.

Third (and perhaps most important), the cases with birthmarks and birth defects provide a better explanation than any other now available about why some persons have birth defects when most persons do not and for why some persons who have a birth defect have theirs in a particular location instead of elsewhere. We need to judge this claim against present knowledge of the causes of birth defects. Research on birth defects has identified several causes of them: genetic factors, certain viral infections, and chemicals (such as thalidomide and alcohol). Yet these and other recognized causes account for less than half of all birth defects. (The figures assigned to birth defects of "unknown causes" vary in different series but range between 43.2% and 70%.)

Even taking account of the identified medical causes, modern medicine has nothing to say about why a particular *person* has a birth defect when another person does not. Indeed, modern medicine, with its reductionist and mechanical approach to illness, rarely recognizes a person as anything more than the behavioral expression of his or her body. From this perspective, there is no person other than the body. Thus, if someone is born with a birth defect, physicians nearly always attribute this to chance. The cases of this work suggest that for some birth defects we can say why a person has a birth defect and why the birth defect is in one location instead of in another.

Scientific publications have a rule that is sound, if austere: An author should not state his or her conclusions before presenting the evidence that supports them. I have departed from this rule because I think my readers need to remember, as they read further, the three different values of the cases with birthmarks and birth defects: They provide objective types of evidence, they suggest the influence of a discarnate personality on a later-born baby, and they help us understand why, in some cases, a person with a birth defect has it at a particular location.

In the preceding paragraphs I have mentioned birth defects more than birthmarks and will now say something further about the latter. Unlike birth defects, nearly everyone has a birthmark. In fact, one survey showed that the average adult has about 15 birthmarks on his or her body. Yet except for a few rare instances of pedigrees showing the inheritance of birthmarks at the same location, nothing is known about why a person has a birthmark at one location instead of another. As with birth defects, the cases of this work suggest an answer to that question, at least for some birthmarks.

Furthermore, most of the birthmarks that I describe differ from the kind of birthmark that almost everyone has. These latter are small areas of increased pigmentation that are called nevi by physicians and moles by most laypeople. Some of the birthmarks of the cases I describe are of this type, but most are not. Instead, they are hairless areas of puckered, scarlike tissue, often raised above surrounding tissues or depressed below them; a few are areas of decreased pigmentation. Some are bleeding or oozing when the baby is born. Those that resemble nevi and moles in appearance are often larger than "ordinary" nevi and also often occur in unusual locations.

The birthmarks and birth defects occur within the context of a case that nearly always has other features. Not all of these figure in every case, and the first that I shall mention is rare. A case may begin when a person—usually an elderly one who believes death is approaching—expresses a wish to be reborn to a particular couple who, the dying person believes, will make good parents. The person may express a further desire to change some physical trait so that in the next life he or she would, for example, be born without flat feet. Predictions of these kinds occur with some frequency among the Tlingit of Alaska and also among the lamas of Tibet. People of other cultures, so far as my experience goes, rarely make them.

The next feature in the development of a case is often a dream or dreams in which a deceased person appears and expresses an intention to be reborn to particular parents. I call these announcing dreams. The dreamer is usually a woman who will be the mother of the baby in whose body the announcing deceased personality intends to reincarnate. Sometimes other members of the family, or even friends, may have announcing dreams. Although such dreams occur in many different cultures, they are particularly prominent features in the cases of the Tlingit of Alaska and the Burmese. The time of their occurrence varies in different cultures. Among the Tlingit, the announcing dream usually occurs just before the *birth* of the child in question. In contrast, among the Burmese the dream nearly always occurs before the *conception* of the child. This accords with the Buddhist belief, at least in Burma (now called Myanmar), that once conception has occurred the deceased personality becomes tied to the developing embryo and can no longer communicate with other persons through dreams. Recognizable announcing dreams rarely occur in the cases of Sri Lanka, the United States (other than the North American tribes), and Lebanon. In Sri Lanka and the United States, there are few "same-family" cases, by which I mean that the subject of the case and the person whose life it will claim to remember belong to the same family. Therefore, if a mother-to-be or other person did have a dream about a discarnate person, the dreamer might not recognize the person dreamed about, and so nothing comprehensible could be announced or remembered. As for Lebanon, the Druses of that country and surrounding countries believe that persons cannot exist incorporeally (until the Day of Judgment). According to their belief, a person is reborn in a new physical body the instant he or she dies; this leaves no time for sending messages in dreams.

A variant of the announcing dream occurs that I call a departing dream. In such a dream, a person who has died appears to a member of his or her family and tells the dreamer in what family he or she will reincarnate or perhaps has already reincarnated. In a few cases, the information thus conveyed has enabled the family of the deceased person to locate and meet the newborn baby said to be the reincarnation of that person.

When a baby is born, its parents will immediately notice any major birth defect. They may, however, overlook birthmarks, especially if they are small. Much depends on the care with which they examine the baby. This, in turn, varies with the importance they give to identifying the baby as a particular person reborn. Some cultures, such as those of the Tlingit of Alaska and the Igbo of Nigeria, attach great importance to such identification. In those cultures, if you had been, for example, a famous warrior or even a successful trader, you can pick up some of your previous prestige as you are reborn—provided, that is, that your parents recognize you for who you were. This may require careful examination of a baby for birthmarks. I remember from my early work in Alaska an elderly

Tlingit totem-pole carver who deplored to me that no one of his tribe any longer knew how to examine babies for birthmarks. He might have been even more disappointed with the Indians of Asia, many of whom do not expect to find birthmarks on babies and may miss many because they do not look for them.

In our investigations of these cases, we require that one or more informed adults testify that he or she noticed the birthmark immediately after the child's birth or, at most, within a few weeks of the birth. Sometimes we have been shown a boy of, say, 8 years of age who had numerous marks on his body, from insect bites, cuts, abrasions, and furuncles, as well as a possible birthmark. The parents have not always been sure which, if any, of these marks was present at the child's birth.

The fourth feature in the development of a case occurs when the child (whom we should now call the subject) begins to speak, or soon afterward. If a child is going to speak about a previous life, it nearly always begins to do so between the ages of 2 and 4. A few may begin earlier and before they have learned to speak coherently. They may mispronounce words and use gestures to communicate what they want to say. At first, what they say may make no sense to the parents, who only understand the child's words when it can enunciate clearly. A few children do not speak until after the age of 4. I studied the case of one child in Lebanon who had some dreams about a previous life when he was about 6, and then said almost nothing about it until he was 12 years old; but he was exceptional.

In most cases the child continues to talk about the previous life until he or she is about 5 to 7 or 8 years old. At this age the memories usually appear to fade. This, however, is a matter difficult to judge, and it seems that some children continue to remember the previous life, but stop speaking about it. They "go underground," as it were. This may happen especially with a girl who could speak loquaciously about having a husband and children up to the age of 8 or 10; but at a later age, the girl would be embarrassed, maybe even compromised, if she continued to talk as if she were a married woman.

Most of the children speak about the previous life with an intensity, even with strong emotion, that surprises the adults around them. Many of them do not at first distinguish past from present, and they may use the present tense in referring to the previous life. They may say, for example: "I *have* a wife and two sons. I *live* in Agra." Although some children make 50 or more different statements, others make only a few but repeat these many times, often tediously. At the other extreme, some children whom adults have identified as a deceased person reborn (perhaps on the basis of dreams or birthmarks) make no statements at all about the previous life with which they are identified.

The content of what the child states nearly always includes some account of the death in the previous life. This is particularly true if the death was violent, but occurs also—less frequently—when it was natural. Beyond that, the child usually speaks about the family of the previous life. Remembering the parents of that life, the child may use some phrase like "my real parents" to distinguish the parents of the previous life from its parents. The child often asks, and frequently importunes, its parents to take it to the previous family. Sooner or later most parents accede to these requests, partly to appease the child and partly to satisfy their own curiosity about the accuracy of what the child has been saying. Critical neighbors who hint that the child is narrating fantasies may further stimulate the child's parents to have it vindicated against such aspersions.

If the child has given sufficient and adequately specific details, especially of proper names and places, it is usually possible to identify a deceased person the facts of whose life closely match the child's statements. (We call this person the "previous personality," a phrase that acknowledges a terrestrial existence while allowing that the personality is no longer tied to a physical body; I may use the term even when no matching deceased person is found, but is only conjectured.) If a previous personality is found whose life corresponds to the child's statements, we speak of the case as "solved." In many cases, however, the child's statements are not sufficiently specific or, for other reasons, no matching person can be found. Such cases are "unsolved." They are difficult to interpret. In many respects they have features similar to those of solved cases, but in the absence of verified details they may be nothing but fantasies.

If the child's parents know or find the family to which the child has been referring and the two families meet, they understandably exchange information about what the child has said and how much of that is correct or wrong. The child may also recognize spontaneously (or on request) various persons, objects, and places known to the previous personality. I attach little importance to these recognitions because of the strong possibility that persons present could give the child cues, albeit without intending to do so. The informants themselves often give the child's recognitions great weight in their appraisal of the case, and I have known informants to reject an entire case because the child—perhaps by then much frightened by a crowd of onlookers—failed to recognize them.

The first three features in the development of a case (if they occur)—prediction of rebirth, announcing dreams, and birthmarks or birth defects—fix in the parents' minds a belief about the identity of the child in its previous life. This entails the risk that they will encourage or even guide the child to speak about the previous life of the person identified. I have known a few cases in which a parent has damaged an otherwise good case by overenthusiastic instigation of the child to speak about the presumed previous life. The best assurance we have against the frequent occurrence of such behavior lies in the comparative indifference of most of the parents (in the Asian countries) to what the child states. If a child has a birth defect, they—believing in reincarnation—attribute the defect to *some* previous life; it does not matter much to them *which* previous life it may have been. Moreover, a substantial number of parents, far from encouraging their children to speak about previous lives, take measures to suppress such expressions. In India, we found that 41% of the parents in a series of cases had done this. The parental measures of suppression have no observable effect. The children nearly always stop speaking about the previous lives (and seem to forget them) between the ages of 5 and 8 whether they are suppressed or not. The endeavors at suppression, however, probably pacify the parents.

There are several motives for such suppressive measures. In India it is widely believed—without any evidence whatever—that children who talk about previous lives are fated to die young. In addition, parents often object to the content of the previous life the child describes. If the parents belong to the middle levels in social and economic terms and the child talks about a previous life in a much higher station, they may not wish to hear the child repeatedly bragging about having many servants and demeaning the clothes and food they are providing for it. Equally unwelcome would be talk about life at a much lower level, such as that of a street-sweeper, or about some sordid murder.

Mention of these last types of statements brings me to the fifth important feature of the cases: the child's unusual behavior, by which I mean behavior that is unusual for the child's family, but harmonious with what can be known or conjectured about the person of whom the child speaks. If the child recalls a previous life in superior social circumstances, it may refuse to participate normally in the life of its family. I have known children of lower caste Indian families who, believing that they had been (and in their view still were) Brahmins, would refuse to eat their family's food, which they considered polluted. Conversely, a child remembering the life of a street-sweeper may show an alarming lack of concern about cleanliness.

Phobias, nearly always related to the mode of death in the previous life, occur in about 35% of the cases. A child remembering a life that ended in drowning may be afraid of being immersed in water; one who remembers a life that ended in shooting may show a phobia of guns and loud noises. If the death occurred during a vehicular accident, the subject may have a phobia of automobiles, buses, and trucks. These phobias often manifest before the child has begun to speak. There is no model for them in other members of the family, and the child has undergone no experience since its birth that could account for the phobia; hence the possibility that it derives from the previous life, as the child, when it can speak, says it does. As with phobias following a trauma in this life, the phobias of these children tend to diminish as they become older.

Philias also occur often. They frequently take the form of a desire or demand for particular foods (not eaten in the subject's family) or for clothes different from those customarily worn by the family members. Under this heading also come instances of cravings for addicting substances, such as tobacco, alcohol, and other drugs that the previous personality was known to have used.

A few subjects show skills that they have not been taught (or sufficiently watched others demonstrating), but which the previous personality was known to have had.

In cases of what we call the "sex-change" type, the child says it remembers a previous life as a person of the opposite sex. Such children almost invariably show traits of the sex of the claimed previous life. They cross-dress, play the games of the opposite sex, and may otherwise show attitudes characteristic of that sex. As with the phobias, the attachment to the sex and habits of the previous life usually becomes attenuated as the child grows older; but a few of these children remain intransigently fixed to the sex of the previous life, and one has become homosexual.

Particularly vivid examples of unusual behavior occur in subjects who claim to remember previous lives as natives of a country different from that of their parents. Examples of subjects of such "international cases" occur often in Burma. We have studied the cases of at least 20 Burmese children—now all adults—who said when they were young that they had been Japanese soldiers killed in Burma during World War II. None gave sufficient details to permit verification of its statements. All, however, showed a number of traits that I call "Japanese." By this I mean that they behaved in ways that were typical of Japanese people (especially Japanese soldiers) at the time of World War II. Such traits include industriousness; insensitivity to pain; complaints about the heat and the spicy food of Burma; and demands for raw fish, sweet foods, and strong sweet tea. (The Burmese drink a weak tea without sugar.) In all these behaviors these children differed markedly from their parents and siblings.

The deaths remembered by the children are predominantly violent. The overall percentage of violent deaths in the previous life is 51%, but the incidence varies (in solved cases) from a low of 29% among the Haida of northwestern North America to a high of 74% in Turkey. These incidences far exceed those of violent death in the general populations of the countries where the cases occur.

As I mentioned, the children usually remember the mode of death in the previous life, especially if it ended violently. And they often remember the other persons concerned in the death—usually murderers. The children often show strong animosities and attitudes of vengefulness toward these persons, especially if they happen to meet them. The animosity may generalize to other members of the same group. For example, a child in India who remembered a previous life that ended in murder by a Moslem might show a hatred for all Moslems.

Many of the children express memories of the previous life in their play. Some children play with other children toward whom they assume the role of the adult person whose life they remember. Thus, a girl who remembered a previous life as a schoolteacher would assemble her playmates as pupils and play at instructing them with an imaginary blackboard. A child who remembered the life of a garage mechanic would spend hours under a family sofa "repairing" the car that it represented for him.

A few children enact in their play the mode of death in the previous life, especially if it ended in suicide. One child who remembered a life that ended in suicidal hanging had the macabre habit of walking around with a piece of rope attached around his neck. Two children who remembered drowning themselves used to play at drowning.

I find it convenient to subsume all the various types of unusual behavior these children show under the collective term "behavioral memory," which distinguishes this kind of memory from the cognitive memories and mental images of events that find expression in the child's statements about the previous life. The behavioral memories, such as phobias and likings for particular foods, often last after the child can no longer remember any of the imaged memories.

Readers may not appreciate from what I have described that remembering a previous life is almost never a pleasant experience. Too often the children are troubled by confusion regarding their identity, and this becomes even more severe in those children who, conscious of being in a small body, can remember having been in an adult one, or who remember a life as a member of the opposite sex. To these tormenting awarenesses may be added a tearing division of loyalties between present and previous families.

The cases of the children who claim to remember previous lives have four features that occur so regularly that I have presumed to call them "universal." These are: the early age of speaking about the previous life (between the ages of 2 and 4); the later age of ceasing to speak about the previous life (usually between the ages of 5 and 8); a high incidence of violent death in the previous life; and frequent mention of the mode of death in the previous life.

Other features vary, sometimes widely, from one culture to another. I have already mentioned the relatively high incidence of announcing dreams in Burma and among the Tlingit of Alaska, and their paucity in the cases of Sri Lanka and the United States (other than tribal groups). Similarly, the incidence of cases of the sex-change type varies widely. In Burma about 26% of cases are of this type, and the percentage of such cases is also high in Nigeria (18%) and Thailand (13%). In India, however, sex-change cases comprise only 3% of the total; and in Lebanon and among the tribes of northwestern North America sex-change cases seem not to occur at all. There is a similar, although narrower range in the median length of the interval between the previous personality's death and the subject's birth. This extends from only 4 months among the Haida of northwestern North America to 34 months among the Igbo of Nigeria.

Our investigation of a case of this type begins as soon as we can reach its scene. Ideally, we would like to arrive there before the two families concerned have met, but this is rarely possible. As I mentioned, we sometimes do not reach the case until months and even years after its development. I have said that the case usually begins when the subject is a young child; but he or she may be an adult before we arrive at the scene of the case. If the subject has a birthmark or birth defect, the case is still worth studying, although it is obvious that the available witnesses will be fewer and their memories of the development of the case probably weaker than those of informants we meet while a case is still fresh. The delay in investigating the older cases partly accounts for the paucity of information that will be found in my reports of some of them (in the monograph).

When we do reach the case—be it early or late—we begin with interviews on the side of the subject and its family. We interview the child (if it will talk with us), its parents, and such other persons as can provide *firsthand* testimony about the child's statements and any unusual behavior it may have shown. These may be older siblings, grandparents, teachers, and other informed persons. We examine, sketch, and photograph the child's birthmarks or birth defects. We ask for any written documents, such as identity cards, diaries, or horoscopes, that may provide exact records of dates.

Next we go to the family of the claimed previous life (if the case is solved) and conduct a series of interviews with members of the family, who must, similarly, be firsthand witnesses of what they describe. A particularly important part of the inquiry is concerned with any previous acquaintance between the two families or the possibility that they had some mutual acquaintance (even if they themselves did not know each other). We want to exclude as well as we can the possibility that the child might have overheard other persons talking about the details concerning the deceased person of whom the child has been speaking.

In the cases with birthmarks and birth defects, we have spared no effort to obtain postmortem reports or other documents that establish the location of the wounds on the deceased person concerned. These records were made before the subject was born and without any thought of their use for our research. The medical documents have great value in themselves. In addition, as I shall explain later, they tend to increase confidence in the accuracy of the testimony of informants for most of the cases for which we have no medical documents.

Ahead of my readers lie 13 chapters—most of them about children who claimed to remember previous lives and who had relevant birthmarks—that they will read before coming to Chapter 15, in which I discuss the several possible interpretations of these cases. These interpretations are the ones that seem most pertinent to me, but there may be others that I have not been able to imagine. I think it will help readers if I summarize these interpretations now. Readers may thus be thinking about them as they study the case reports ahead.

One must first be adequately confident about the authenticity of each case. Is the account given here an adequate report of what actually happened? Whenever I think of the word *authenticity*, I remember that informants tried to recall events that happened weeks, months, and sometimes years before they spoke with me. Their memories were imperfect and their biases often obscure. With rare exceptions they spoke to me through interpreters; the interpreters tried their best to give a full translation, but inevitably something was lost, or perhaps distorted. My note-taking, even after many years of practice, was imperfect. Next, when writing the case reports I had to select from my field notes what to include in a published report. (A second selection occurred in the preparation of this synopsis; but I have already exhorted readers to reach no firm judgment without studying its parent monograph.) Given these important sources of error, what defenses do we have against them? There are several. First, whenever I could, I obtained the testimony of several informants whose statements I could compare. Second, I had the good fortune, for most cases, to have interpreters who worked with me for many years and who shared my interest in exactitude. Finally, the cases, even of widely separated cultures, show some similar features. I must admit, however, that in the end the reader has to accept my assertion that I would not have published these case reports unless I believed that they are authentic. This does not mean that I claim all details are accurate, only that what the reader can examine corresponds adequately to events that happened.

Given the authenticity of the cases, what are the next steps toward a rational explanation of them? We must first consider normal explanations. Among these there is the possibility that the child's family had mistakenly identified a deceased person whose wounds happened—just by chance—to correspond, more or less, to birthmarks on their child. They then decided that their child was the reincarnation of this deceased person; and they encouraged the child to think this also, until the child came to believe it. All this could be entirely innocent; but it can happen. I have described elsewhere one case (Kenedi Alkan) that developed in this way, and there may be a few others not known to me. I do not think there can be more than a few. I say this partly because the parents—surprising as this may be to many Western readers—are often slow to identify their child with a deceased person; and partly because the correspondence between wounds and birthmarks and the child's correct statements about the life of the deceased person usually leave no doubt that the correct previous personality has been identified.

Suppose that we find an indisputable correspondence between wounds on a deceased person and birthmarks (and other features, such as statements) of a child. How shall we explain the correspondence? Suppose further that the two families had no knowledge of each other before the case developed. We now have to consider what are called paranormal interpretations. The first of these is that the correspondence between birthmarks on the child and wounds on the identified deceased person have occurred by chance and that the child has obtained the information included in its correct statements about the deceased person by extrasensory perception. The principal difficulty with this interpretation is that the children concerned in these cases show no ability for extrasensory perception of the kind required in most cases, except in connection with their claimed memories.

A second paranormal explanation supposes that a discarnate personality controls or "possesses" the subject and imposes memories of its life on the child. This interpretation does not explain the almost invariable fading or amnesia of the child's apparent memories between the ages of 5 and 8 years. Why should possessing personalities all withdraw their influence, as it were, when children are at about the same age? This interpretation also does not explain the birthmarks, unless we suppose that the possession occurs before the child's birth. We then may ask how this situation would differ from reincarnation.

A third paranormal explanation supposes that the child's mother, knowing about the deceased person's wounds, somehow reproduces them on her baby. This is the process known as a maternal impression, and I shall give examples of it and discuss it in Chapter 3. Suffice it to say here that such a process entails that the mother would also impose the principal features of the concerned deceased person's personality on the child, so that it would identify with that person and utter statements apparently derived from the person's memories of his or her life. I find this explanation plausible to a certain extent. It could not, however, apply to 25 cases that I have investigated in which the child's mother had no knowledge of the deceased person's wounds. It also supposes that the mothers have more time, inclination, and ability to impose an identification on a child than I think they have.

If we reject all the foregoing interpretations and can think of no other, we may consider reincarnation the best one. We should not decide that it is the best however, until we have carefully appraised and rejected the others. I will repeat and amplify these interpretations in Chapter 15.

I do not expect my readers to accept readily the idea that the mind of a dead person can influence the form of a later-born baby. In order to make this idea easier to assimilate, I describe in the next two chapters ways in which images in the mind of a living person may produce local changes in that person's own body and, less often, in the body of another living person. After these two chapters I turn to the descriptions of the birthmarks corresponding to wounds (or other marks) on deceased persons.

I will conclude this chapter now with a few remarks about my presentations of the case reports, which will avoid later unnecessary repetitions or digressions in the text.

In its statements the child is expressing what certainly seem to it to be memories. This may not be the view, at least initially, of its parents, and it may not be that of my readers. It would, however, be tedious for me to keep reminding my readers that I am referring to "claimed memories" or "seeming memories." I have therefore often omitted such qualifying words as *ostensible, claimed,* and so on. This does not mean that I intend to beg the main question of this research, which is whether the claimed memories are real memories or have some other explanation. By *real memories* I mean mental images that correspond to events that other informants say occurred.

When I describe a birthmark or birth defect on a subject, it should be understood that—with rare exceptions—no one else in the child's family has a similar abnormality. In the few cases in which the subject and previous personality belong to the same family and a genetic factor might account for the subject's abnormality, I will mention this possibility.

Unless I note exceptions, the families concerned in the cases in India are Hindus; those of Sri Lanka, Burma, and Thailand are Theravadan Buddhists; those of Turkey are Alevis (a Shiite sect of Islam); and those of Lebanon are Druses. The Igbos of Nigeria and the natives of Alaska and British Columbia are usually Christians formally; but they nearly all adhere more or less to their traditional religions, which include the belief in reincarnation.

In 1989, the name of the country called Burma was changed to Myanmar, and the name of its capital, Rangoon, was changed to Yangon. Some other place-names in this country were also changed. Because all the cases in this country were investigated before 1989, I have used the old names in the case reports. In Burma, honorifics, like *Maung, U, Ma,* and *Daw,* are so important and used so regularly by the Burmese that they seem almost part of a person's name; accordingly, I have used them in front of the Burmese names.

2

BODILY CHANGES CORRESPONDING TO MENTAL IMAGES IN THE PERSON AFFECTED

The bleeding wounds known as stigmata on the hands, feet, chest, and (sometimes) other parts of the body are among the best known and least understood of abnormal bodily changes. Different writers have attributed them all to sanctity, to hysteria, and to malingering (that is, self-inflicted wounding). As generalizations, these opinions are all incorrect. A few instances of persons wounding themselves, usually from zealous identification with Jesus, have been exposed. In the great majority of cases, however, we can confidently exclude artifactual wounding; many of the subjects have been under close surveillance, and in a few cases observers have actually watched stigmata (or at least the bleeding) develop before their eyes.

St. Francis of Assisi was the first notable person to develop stigmata. His wounds came on toward the end of a long period of about 40 days that he spent by himself, during which he was entirely absorbed in contemplating the Passion of Jesus. (His stigmata were also among the most unusual ever observed in that protrusions somewhat in the form of clenched nails were said to have come out of his wounds.) In the seven and a half centuries following St. Francis's death, about 350 cases of stigmatists have been recorded. The stigmatists were nearly all religious persons, such as nuns, and a few were saints; St. Catherine of Siena and St. Gemma Galgani were two of these. St. Catherine of Siena had a vision of Jesus with his wounds and with rays of light running from them to her body. Her stigmata then occurred at the sites of her body where the rays seen coming from Jesus impinged on her.

Until the second half of the 19th century nearly all writers about stigmata believed them to be the result of a special grace bestowed on saints or saintlike persons. The attribution of saintliness thus might be given retrospectively to someone who developed stigmata; whoever had stigmata must be saintly.

In the second half of the 19th century, some early psychologists began to study what we now call psychosomatic relationships and came to view stigmata as illustrating these. They were in the first instance encouraged in this interpretation because nearly all the authenticated cases of stigmata had occurred in women. Women were notoriously more liable than men to develop what was then called *hysteria*, which was being understood with increasing clarity as a psychosomatic disorder in which beliefs about the body become expressed in changes in bodily functions. (Young women of child-bearing age are more hypnotizable—therefore more suggestible— than men or than women of other ages.) Then it was noted that some stigmatists, although pious in their ways, were far from being saints. Furthermore, the stigmata varied greatly in form, size, appearance, and even location. Nearly all stigmatists showed wounds at the feet, hands, and lower chest. Three stigmatists were credibly reported to have developed marks and deep indentations around the wrists as they relived the scene when Jesus was arrested and bound with ropes; the marks on the stigmatists' wrists seemed to reproduce the marks that binding ropes would make. (I ask readers to remember these last cases when I describe in later chapters children who had ropelike birthmarks that informants attributed to ropes binding the previous personalities shortly before they died.) Readers should also note the case described later in this chapter, the ropelike marks of which are shown in Figure 1.

The stigmatists' chest wounds showed important variations. Some of them had the chest wound on the left side and some had it on the right. The Bible does not say into which side of Jesus a Roman soldier thrust his spear; and because there was only one spear thrust recorded, right or left may be correct, but both cannot be. Such variations strongly suggested that stigmata were bodily changes produced by the mental images of the stigmatist.

There was other pertinent evidence. Some of the stigmata bore a close relationship to the wounds on the representation—for example, a statuette—of Jesus before which the stigmatist was accustomed to worship. An early 19th-century stigmatist had on her chest a Y-shaped lesion that matched an unusual Y-shaped crucifix in the church where she worshipped. And the biographer of another stigmatist (of the late 19th century) remarked on the close correspondence between the stigmatist's wounds and those on the statuette of Jesus before which this saint worshipped.

In the 1920s, a German physician had the good fortune to find a young girl—a Protestant—who easily went into deep hypnosis. This girl (Elisabeth K.) had a high degree of impressionability. She attended a slide show that vividly depicted the sufferings of Jesus as he was led to the cross and crucified. On the following day the girl complained of severe pain in her hands and feet (at the sites of the nails driven into Jesus' limbs). The physician, seizing this opportunity, hypnotized the girl and told her to imagine that nails were being driven deeply into her hands and feet. The next day the girl had open wounds at these places (*). Subsequently, the physician readily induced in this girl simulacra of Jesus' other wounds, including those of a crown of thorns complete with triangle-shaped lesions (*), similar to wounds that thorns might make.

None of this newer evidence or revised appraisal of old evidence need detract from the reputation for sanctity that the great majority of stigmatists had and deserved. It does, however, undermine the idea that stigmata are a grace vouchsafed only to the elect. What then is the role of sanctity in the occurrence of stigmata? I suggest that the connection occurs through the concentration of the mind on particular parts of the body. Many saintly persons are almost fully absorbed in the life and death of Jesus and determined to be as much like him as they possibly can. It is difficult for the ordinary person to understand the intense identification with Jesus that some of them have achieved. In doing so, their concentration on his wounds acts to produce similar lesions in themselves. I do not mean to say that concentration is the only factor of importance in the occurrence of stigmata; but before returning to this topic I shall describe some other examples of the effects mental images may have on local bodily functions.

A mother sometimes develops imitative or "sympathetic" pains at the same location as her child has a pain, say from a toothache. Sometimes the imitative effects go beyond pain and include visible changes in the tissues affected. For example, one mother watching her little son at play saw a heavy window sash fall on his hand and crush three of his fingers. She immediately felt severe pain in the same fingers that had been injured in her son; and afterward her fingers became swollen and inflamed so that pus developed in them and had to be evacuated.

Hypnosis is not a state that I wish or need to define. It depends, in the first place, on the replacement of ideas in the mind of the subject with ideas in the mind of the hypnotist. This is what we mean by suggestion. Once the subject accepts the initial ideas of the hypnotist, he or she enters a state of increasing susceptibility to further suggestions offered by the hypnotist. In this way the hypnosis can be "deepened" and the subject also enabled to go into hypnosis more readily at the next occasion. Another important feature of hypnosis is heightened concentration of the mind. Hypnosis also facilitates the links between mental images and bodily functions that the images may influence. It greatly lubricates, so to say, the psychophysiological processes of the body.

We have no understanding at present of the mind's ability to select and influence the right processes in order to carry out a suggestion given during hypnosis. Consider our physical experience when we become thirsty. A dryness of the mouth leads us to describe ourselves as thirsty and needing more fluid. Already, however, the body will have made its own adjustments by reducing the excretion of water in the urine. This entails modifying the release of a certain hormone from the pituitary gland, the one that controls water excretion. Now let a person who is not dehydrated and not thirsty be hypnotized and told that he or she *is* thirsty. Soon his or her kidneys will diminish the excretion of urine just as they would if he or she had been dehydrated. Somehow the body has picked out the right hormone (or perhaps some other link in the process of urine formation) and implemented a decrease in the excretion of urine.

Hypnosis has been used to modify a wide variety of bodily functions through the offering of appropriate instructions to a hypnotized person. The heart rate can be slowed or speeded up. Bleeding can be stopped and menstruation started at certain times. Breasts can be enlarged. Anesthesia can be induced, including an unusual type of anesthesia known as "glove and stocking anesthesia." This phrase refers to the abrupt line of demarcation at the upper end of the induced anesthesia, a line that does not correspond to the distribution of the nerves serving the arms and legs, but corresponds instead to the idea implanted in the subject's mind. (Glove and stocking anesthesia may also occur spontaneously in persons who give themselves this idea of what an area of anesthesia is like.) There is a rare condition called *oedème bleu* in which an arm becomes swollen, painful, bluish, and of little use. It may follow some relatively minor injury to the arm that concentrates the patient's attention on it. In the 19th century *oedème bleu* was induced and removed with hypnosis.

Between about 1880 and 1930 a large number of experiments were conducted to study the induction of blisters on the skin of hypnotized subjects. To indicate the proposed site for the blister, the hypnotist would sometimes touch the subject at the place with some object, usually a cold one. The subject was told, or led to believe, that he or she was being burned. Many subjects responded with a blister at the indicated site, as if they had been burned. Some of the early experiments were insufficiently rigorous in that the patient was not kept under surveillance, so that he or she might have scratched the indicated site in an effort to comply with the hypnotist's suggestion. Most experiments have avoided this mistake, however, and I believe that the evidence is strong enough to convince all but the most resolute skeptics that the phenomenon is genuine.

Most of the experimenters who induced blisters during hypnosis used a small stimulus of no unusual form—such as the tip of the finger—with which to touch the subject at the site where the blister was to occur. A few, however, applied stimuli in the form of letters of the alphabet (or some other unusual form), and the ensuing marks reproduced the recognizable form of the stimulus.

One experimenter thought that blisters induced during hypnosis might occur only if the subject had previously been burned at the site where blisters were to appear. I do not believe that any evidence supports this assertion as a generalization, although a previous burn at a particular site may facilitate the occurrence of inflammation and blisters suggested at the same site.

The examples I have given of bodily changes induced with hypnosis are largely derived from experimental demonstrations of the range and power of hypnosis. The changes in bodily function during hypnosis that I have mentioned cannot be induced in everyone. For many of the effects demonstrated, we now have other and quicker means of bringing about the results obtained, if we want them. For example, chemical anesthesia is superior to hypnosis for surgical operations.

Hypnosis, however, still has an important role to play in relieving pain. It may also be of great value in some intractable skin diseases. For example, warts have been successfully removed with hypnosis. Moreover, they may be removed from one area at a time, another demonstration of how the mind somehow finds the right part of the body for executing the instructions given. A particularly impressive improvement in a skin disease occurred when a hypnotist successfully treated a patient with intractable ichthyosis ("fish-scale disease"). He treated his patient limb by limb with improvements occurring successively in each limb as it was indicated by the suggestions offered.

The intense revival of memories of some earlier physical trauma may be accompanied by the appearance of wounds that closely resemble the original wounds. (It may be difficult to be precise about the resemblance if no firsthand observer of the original wounds is available to compare them to the later wounds accompanying the revived memories.) In the 1950s, several examples of this phenomenon were published. In one of the most impressive, the subject relived (with the help of ether) an occasion when, being in a hospital and requiring restraint, his arms had been tied with a rope. When the patient relived this experience, deep curved depressions appeared on his lower arms. They were exactly like those that occur on the flesh of a person tied with a rope (Figure 1). (I ask readers also to remember this case when I present, later in this work, the cases of persons with birthmarks that informants attributed to marks made by ropes that had tied the previous personality before he or she was killed.) In another published case a patient relived a severe caning inflicted on her by a sadistic father. He had used a carved cane, and the unusual pattern of the carving on the cane appeared on the skin of the patient as she relived being beaten with this cane.

No case of this kind has come under my direct observation. Two psychiatric colleagues of mine, however, sent me written accounts of cases they had observed. In both instances, the patients relived—one with LSD and one with hypnosis—memories of severe beatings. And in both cases, during the reliving, clearly visible marks—actual wheals in one case—appeared at the places where the patients said they had been beaten.

A rare type of physical change corresponding to a mental image sometimes occurs in the experiences of persons in India who come close to death and survive. After regaining consciousness, some of them say that they were mistakenly seized by messengers of the King of the Dead and taken to the "realm of the dead." With discovery of the mistake, they were sent back. Upon recovery, some of these subjects state that they were burned while in the realm of the dead, and they show areas of inflammation or scarring at the sites of the burning. The subject (Durga Jatav) of one of the most bizarre cases of this kind that I have encountered said that he resisted being dragged from life by the messengers of the King of the Dead. He struggled so much that in desperation the messengers cut off his legs at the knees. When the registrar (in the place to which he had been taken) exposed their mistake, they said that he could return; but he then asked to have his legs replaced. Somehow he was refitted with legs and sent back to terrestrial life. He regained consciousness in the bed where his family believed he had died. The remarkable feature of the case was the presence on this man's knees of large scar-like lines closely resembling scars that might occur after horizontal cuts with a knife (*). We obtained X-ray photographs of the patient's knees, but these showed no abnormality.

I shall now discuss what I consider the common factors underlying most, if not all, of the bodily changes that I have described in this chapter. Violence is the first of these. Readers will have noticed the prominent part that violence and physical injury have played in the spontaneously occurring cases. This is certainly true of stigmatism, in which the subject's attention becomes closely focused on the ordeal of Jesus' crucifixion. Physical injury is also prominent in the cases of the recurrence of wounds with the revival of memories of traumatic beatings or restraint. It also enters into the experiments with blisters induced during hypnosis, in which the subject believes he or she is being burned. Violence and the threat of injury are concentrators of attention. I wish to bring them forward here because of the high frequency of violent death, which I mentioned in Chapter 1, among the cases with birthmarks and birth defects related to previous lives. Violence is not, however, the only concentrator of attention. Indeed, stigmatists concentrate on Jesus out of love for him and only secondarily become involved in the violence of his death.

At least two other important factors must enter into the production of physical changes corresponding to mental images. One is a factor of impressionability, now often called absorption. Highly impressionable subjects quickly "lose" themselves in a scene viewed or imagined. If someone calls their name, they seem not to hear and do not respond. Many persons would have seen the slide show of Jesus' crucifixion without being affected as was Elisabeth K., who so readily developed stigmata at the site of Jesus' wounds; they lacked her capacity for absorption.

The third factor we must consider is the reactivity of the tissues of the skin. Persons vary widely in the sensitivity of their skins to stimuli. For example, 25% of persons who are firmly stroked on the skin with a blunt instrument will develop a definite flare around the area stroked, and 5% will show a wheal where the stroking instrument passed over the skin; but the rest will show nothing. It is sometimes possible to write letters on the skin (of the back, for example) of the sensitive patients; this condition is called dermographism, and I will describe an example of paranormal dermographism in the next chapter.

Another example of varying reactivity of the skin occurs in the formation of the dense, indurated scars known as keloids. These occur much more often in some persons than in others and more often in some races, such as Africans, than in others.

I do not mean this list of factors to be exhaustive; there may, for example, be subtle differences in the central and autonomic nervous systems that mediate control of the blood vessels of the skin, and these may play an important part in the changes with which we are here concerned.

A formula that might represent the principal factors would be:

$$CA + DI + PF = CS$$

where CA stands for Concentrated Attention or Absorption, DI for Duration of the Imagery, PF for the hypothetical Physiological Factor (or Factors), and CS for the resultant Changes in the Skin. Although this formula looks simple, I intend it to underscore the complexity of the subject and the deficiencies in our understanding of how physical changes corresponding to mental images occur.

I wish to emphasize that many of the physical changes I have described do not correspond to known configurations of nerves or blood vessels of the skin. I already mentioned this discrepancy in connection with glove and stocking anesthesia. It is equally true of the lesions of stigmatists and of blisters induced by hypnotic suggestion. Concerning the last-named phenomenon, some years ago a leading expert on hypnosis carefully reviewed the literature on such experiments and came near to concluding that the phenomenon must be genuine. He pulled himself back, however, because, he wrote, the occurrence of such blisters makes no sense in relation to the known distribution of the nerves and blood vessels of the skin. He is not the first scientist to deny facts discordant with his assumptions, but he does deserve credit for his candor. The term *paranormal* seems to fit phenomena such as stigmata and hypnotically induced physiological changes. It explains nothing, but has the merit of not denying the occurrence of phenomena for which we have as yet no satisfying explanation.

3

BODILY CHANGES CORRESPONDING TO ANOTHER PERSON'S MENTAL IMAGES

In the preceding chapter I concluded that some paranormal process must occur between the mental images in a person's mind and the production on his or her body of wounds, such as stigmata or blisters induced during hypnosis, the shapes of which have no relationship to the anatomical distribution of the blood vessels or nerves of the skin. Future research may someday show presently undiscovered patterns of nerves and blood vessels that could account for the correspondence between mental images and local bodily changes in the person having the images. Even so, we should still need the word *paranormal* in trying to understand how mental images in one person's mind may affect changes in *another* person's body. This chapter is about such changes.

The simplest examples occur as variants of what I call telepathic impressions. The word *telepathy* means communication between minds without the known sensory organs. In many instances of telepathy the percipient obtains substantial information, perhaps in the form of a visual representation, about the circumstances of another person, called the target person or agent. (The word *sender*, sometimes used for this person, is not so helpful, because the agent often plays no conscious active role in the communication.) In the variant of telepathy called telepathic impressions, almost no content is conveyed, only an impression that, say, someone known to the percipient needs help. Occasionally, a little more detail may be included, such as that the agent is in a hospital; and sometimes less detail is included. For example, a traveler away from home may feel unexpectedly impelled to turn around and go back because something is "wrong at home"; but the percipient does not know *what* is wrong there or who needs help. In a variant of the telepathic impression the percipient has a pain (or sometimes another physical symptom) that corresponds to a pain (or other symptom) in the agent. Here are three examples, the first from the 19th century, the second and third from my own investigations. I give more details of these three cases in my book *Telepathic Impressions.*

A woman awakened one morning with the impression of having received a sharp blow on the mouth. Without understanding this she dressed and went down to breakfast. Her husband, who had been out sailing, joined her. She noticed that he kept dabbing at his mouth with a handkerchief and asked him what he was doing. He then explained that while he had been sailing a gust of wind had suddenly come up, and before he could get out of the way the tiller struck him on the mouth, causing his lip to bleed. This had happened at almost the exact time his wife had awakened with the sense of being struck in the mouth.

In a case that I investigated, an American housewife and mother one morning suddenly experienced a sharp pain in her right leg and buttocks. She was startled and, although she was alone, she said "Oh." Somehow she identified her pain with some trouble to one of her children, who were then away at school. When they came home, she asked them whether anything unusual had happened to them at school. Her 10-year-old daughter then said that while she was playing in the school yard, a boy on a bicycle had run into her and hit her on the backside. She had cried "Oh." As nearly as they could tell, the daughter had been hit at the same time that her mother had had her unexpected pain at the same location.

My third example involved twin sisters. One was in Pennsylvania and known to be pregnant; but she was thought to be in good health, and her delivery was not imminent. Her twin sister was in Naples, Italy, with her husband, a physician. The sister in Italy suddenly developed severe pain in her chest and upper abdomen, with shortness of breath. Her husband could find no signs of physical illness to account for these symptoms. They later learned that her sister in Pennsylvania had gone into labor prematurely and had developed serious complications at the time she was having her symptoms. The twin in Pennsylvania suffered from pain in her chest and shortness of breath, apparently due to a clot in a vein that had broken loose and lodged in her lungs (pulmonary embolus).

Cases of this type require careful appraisal of their details. If we are to consider seriously the interpretation of such a case as an instance of telepathic impression, the temporal coincidence between the symptoms of the two participants must be exact or extremely close; the symptoms must be identical or closely similar and in the same organs or regions of the body; and finally, we must be confident that the percipient had no normal means of learning about or inferring the agent's symptoms before his or hers occurred. I believe the three cases I described meet these criteria.

Mediums, who are persons apparently able to communicate with discarnate personalities, occasionally take on the symptoms of a communicator's fatal illness. In one published case of this kind, the medium began to choke and cough as she described the death of a communicator from heart disease. (Patients with what is called congestive heart failure frequently cough.) The medium had no normal knowledge of the communicator's mode of death. In another case, a medium developed symptoms in a knee when she handled a glove that belonged to a young woman who had injured her knee in a bicycle accident and continued to have pain there. The sensitive knew nothing of this accident or symptom.

Olga Kahl, a Russian clairvoyant living in France during the 1920s, provided some of the most impressive evidence of the representation of mental images in one person by bodily changes in another. Before describing the standard experiments involving her, I should mention that she showed extreme impressionability, even as a child and young adult. On one occasion she misplaced a string of pearls; the loss preoccupied her, and while the pearls were missing, she developed round areas of redness on the skin of her arms which suggested the form of the missing pearls. On another occasion, when living in Istanbul, she watched a group of dervishes, one of whom pushed a skewer through his cheek; the next day she developed an abscess of the cheek at the corresponding site where the dervish had pushed the skewer through.

Olga Kahl's experimental routine provided for a visitor or experimenter to write (hidden from her) a name or perhaps a design on a small piece of paper. The visitor rolled the piece of paper into a ball, which he kept in his hand without showing it to Olga Kahl. After a short interval, the name or design would appear on the skin of Olga Kahl's arm (sometimes on her upper chest) (*). The letters would stand out in red, evidently from extremely localized changes in the superficial blood vessels. Sometimes a letter of a name was omitted, but then a space would be left for it, as if at some level Olga Kahl was aware of the entire word. Olga Kahl sometimes facilitated the process of her kind of dermographism by rubbing the part of her body where the letters were to appear; but such rubbing covered the entire area affected, and no one ever observed Olga Kahl in any endeavor to scratch the words on her skin. (In the last chapter I described dermographism, but that of Olga Kahl involved no actual tracing of letters on her skin.)

Some of the leading French and English scientists who studied such phenomena during the 1920s investigated Olga Kahl. All expressed themselves fully satisfied that her dermographism was genuine. I am not asserting that the mental image in the mind of the experimenter (who wrote the word or design on a piece of paper) directly influenced Olga Kahl's skin. Perhaps her mind obtained a copy, so to speak, of the experimenter's mental image and reproduced that on her skin. At times, she seemed to know what the target word was before it appeared on her skin, but at other times she did not.

The most widespread evidence of the effect of one person's mental images on the body of another living person occurs in cases of what are generally called maternal impressions. This is the phrase used to designate the supposed causal connection between some event that shocks or frightens a pregnant woman and a defect in her later-born baby. A typical case—a published one—is that of a pregnant woman who happened to see on the street a man with partly amputated feet. She became distressed and began to fear that her baby would be born with similar defects. In fact, it was; parts of its feet were absent, and the defects in its feet corresponded to the ones on the man its mother had seen.

The reality of maternal impressions is accepted in most parts of the world today. It was accepted without challenge in the West until the early 18th century. Advances in anatomy and physiology then showed that there is no physical connection between a pregnant woman and her gestating baby through the placenta or otherwise that could mediate the expression in the baby of a mental image in the mother-to-be. The skepticism that these observations stimulated spread slowly. In the 19th century and through the first two decades of this one, the leading medical journals of the United States, Great Britain, and Europe published numerous reports of maternal impressions. Occasionally, a dissident voice would draw attention to the fact that some or many women were frightened when pregnant, expected to have a malformed baby, but then delivered a normal one. On the other side, one 19th-century author pointed out that the absence of any nervous or other known connection between the mother and child signified nothing, because of the possibility that "mind does in some mysterious way operate across matter." (This admirable refusal to deny phenomena because we cannot explain them foreshadowed the beginnings in 1882 of the scientific study of paranormal phenomena by more than 30 years.)

In 1890 a pediatrician of the University of Virginia reviewed 90 cases of maternal impressions that had been published between 1853 and 1886. He concluded that in 69 (77%) of the 90 cases there was "quite a close correspondence" between the impression upon the mother and her baby's defect. He, too, was aware of the growing skepticism about such cases and commented that "thinking men came to doubt the truth of those things which they could not understand."

I decided to review the evidence for maternal impressions. In doing this, I read reports of approximately 300 cases in medical journals, books, and other publications of the United States, Great Britain, France, Germany, Italy, Holland, and Belgium. From these I selected 50 cases for a detailed analysis. I chose cases in which the correspondence between the stimulus to the pregnant woman and the baby's defect was close. I also chose cases in which both the stimulus to the mother and the defect were unusual. As an example of the latter I mention the case of a woman whose brother had to have his penis amputated for removal of a cancer. While she was pregnant, her curiosity impelled her to have a look at the site of her brother's amputation; she afterward gave birth to a male baby without a penis. I have obtained figures for the incidence of some birth defects in the general population, and that for congenital absence of the penis is 1 in 30,000,000. Other birth defects figuring in these cases are more common, but most are rare or even extremely rare.

An unexpected finding of my analysis of these cases was the discovery that the seemingly causative stimulus to the mother occurred much more often than would be expected by chance in the 1st trimester than in the 2nd and 3rd ones. It seems likely that pregnant women would be equally liable to be exposed to some frightening stimulus at any month of a pregnancy; this observation therefore suggests that susceptibility of the embryo is one important factor in maternal impressions. The 1st trimester is also the one during which the embryo is most sensitive to noxious drugs, such as thalidomide, and to viral infections, such as rubella (German measles).

Some further useful information emerged from my analysis. In more than half the cases, the woman was closely involved with the wounding of another person—an eyewitness, perhaps—or was wounded herself. These woundings acted as the stimulus for the maternal impression. The duration of the woman's exposure to the stimulus seems to have had little effect on the occurrence of a maternal impression. In at least two cases, a woman's fear did not quite match her curiosity about some wound, so she just peeked for an instant at the wound; but that sufficed. Most of the women became "shocked" or "frightened" by the stimulus. Some forgot about it quickly, others became obsessively preoccupied with it and could not stop thinking about it. Some of the women were afraid their babies would be affected, others were not, and a few were (mistakenly) confident that their babies would be normal. The beliefs of the women concerned about the effect on the baby had almost no predictive value.

I have been able to investigate seven cases of maternal impressions of different types and will summarize two of them here.

The mother of the first subject (Calvin Ewing) was a Tlingit of Alaska named Sylvia Ewing. She was born with a small hole—in medical terms, a sinus—near the inner corner of her right eye. This was immediately recognized as a defect corresponding to a chronic stye at the same place from which a deceased relative had suffered. On the basis of this correspondence, an announcing dream, and some evidence from Sylvia's behavior, she was identified as the reincarnation of this relative. Hers was a straightforward case of the reincarnation type, although a somewhat weak one with regard to the strength of the evidence. (I give a detailed report of her case in the monograph.) In childhood, Sylvia suffered a certain amount of discomfort from the sinus, which discharged fluid, especially if she had a cold. She also underwent cruel teasing about the defect from her schoolmates.

In due course Sylvia grew up and married. When she became pregnant, she began to fear that her baby would have a defect like hers. She told me: "I was afraid he would look like me. That is all I thought about—whether he would look like me." Her husband confirmed her statement by saying: "She was always worrying about whether the baby would have a hole in the eye like hers."

After the baby was born and brought to Sylvia, the first place she examined was his eye "to see if he had a hole." He had, and it was at exactly the site of her own—near the inner end of the right eye.

Unlike his mother, this baby boy was not identified as the reincarnation of a deceased relative or of anyone else. There were no identifiable causative factors other than the mother's fear of the reproduction of her defect in her child.

The correspondence between the two defects in this case was exceedingly close both in location and size. Figure 2 shows a photograph of the child's sinus, which can be compared with a photograph of the mother's sinus (*).

In the second case, a male baby (Sampath Priyasantha) was born in Sri Lanka without any arms and with severely deformed legs (*). One of my assistants learned about these unusual defects and sent me a photograph of the baby. I decided to investigate the case as soon as I could, but by the time I was able to reach Sampath Priyasantha's village he had died. He had been able to crawl about a little and was just beginning to speak when he died at the age of about 20 months. He had said nothing about a previous life.

The village was somewhat remote, and having taken the trouble to reach it I decided to ask a few questions. From other cases that I had studied—and that I describe later in this book—it occurred to me that Sampath might have been the reincarnation of someone known to his family who had died after having his arms badly injured, perhaps in an industrial accident. I therefore asked the baby's father whether he knew of anyone who had died after having his arms injured. "Yes," he replied. "There was a man I killed by cutting off his arms and legs with a sword." He then went on to tell me how this had happened. The murdered man was a young ruffian of the village, a notorious bully, and a member of a family given to violence. (The brother of this man told me that he had personally killed three of the family's enemies; they had lost their father when a bomb that he was preparing dropped from his hands and blew him to pieces.) A quarrel broke out over a dog belonging to the bully's family that had come onto the property of Sampath's father and eaten some food. Sampath's father decided to finish with the offensive young man. Without much difficulty, he and his brother got him drunk and lured him over to their side of the village. They then cut off his arms and legs and left him to die. (I obtained a postmortem report in this case, and, with some discrepancies, it confirmed the murderer's account of what he had done; limbs were described as "dangling," not totally severed.)

The murdered man's mother was enraged at her son's death. She repeatedly cursed the murderer and his family, saying that they would be punished for killing her son by having a defective child. (Informants differed as to exactly what she said in cursing the family, but the baby's mother definitely thought the angry mother had specified that she would have a defective child.)

The murderers were arrested and sentenced to imprisonment. The father could come home sometimes on leave, and his wife had another baby, a normal female. The parents thought they had perhaps neutralized the curse. Then the dreadfully malformed Sampath Priyasantha was born, and they realized that perhaps they had not.

The villagers we interviewed for this case were divided between those who believed that Sampath Priyasantha was the reincarnation of the murdered man and those who believed he was simply sent to the murderer's family as punishment for the murder they had committed. In particular, the murdered man's mother could not accept the possibility that her son, who had "done nothing" in her view, should be condemned, if reborn, to a life in a defective body. In view of her curse of the murderer's family, a maternal impression remains a plausible interpretation of the case, but it is unlikely that we shall ever be able to reach a firm conclusion on the matter.

I have devoted more than half of this chapter to maternal impressions because readers should remember this phenomenon as they consider the best interpretation for the cases in succeeding chapters. In most of them, the child's mother knew about or had even seen the wounds on the deceased person whose life the child (usually) claimed to remember when it could speak. So we need to ask whether the correspondences in these cases could have arisen from maternal impressions instead of through some other paranormal process, including reincarnation. This explanation could not apply in some 25 cases in which the mother did not see or know about the wounds on the deceased person; but it could certainly be relevant in many other cases.

4

BIRTHMARKS RELATED TO PREVIOUS LIVES WITHOUT VERIFICATION OF POSSIBLE CORRESPONDING WOUNDS

Although it may seem perverse to present weaker before stronger cases, I do so with the intention of helping readers to become acquainted with the wide range of birthmarks that occur in these cases. In none of the nine cases of the group that I describe here was the presumably related wound on the previous personality observed by any informant. Indeed, for most of the cases such a person was not even identified from the child's statements, so these cases remain unsolved. Nevertheless, the subjects all showed some or much behavior that was unusual in their family but that plausibly accorded with what the subjects said about the previous lives they claimed to remember. A few of the subjects said they remembered events between death in the previous life and their birth.

The first 3 subjects of the group were all Burmese children who said that they remembered previous lives as Japanese soldiers who were killed in Burma. (This sets the dates of death in the presumed previous lives as not later than the spring of 1945, when the British Army conclusively defeated the Japanese Army; Rangoon [now Yangon] was captured early in May 1945.)

U Tinn Sein, the first of these subjects, had a single birthmark on his chest. It was a flat round area of increased pigmentation (*). (Unlike most of the birthmarks of these subjects, which I said were not simple moles or nevi, his was just that.) U Tinn Sein described how in the previous life he, a Japanese soldier, had been near a lake outside the town in Upper Burma where he was born. An airplane had come over the town and, strafing the area with bullets, hit him in the chest. After dying, he said, he remained as a discarnate personality in the area of the lake. For diversion he sometimes frightened persons who walked that way by throwing stones at them. (This was a claim of poltergeist activity from the perspective of a discarnate agent.) After the devastation of the war, firewood was scarce in the town, and U Tinn Sein's future father came out to the area of the lake with a wagon to collect firewood. The discarnate Japanese soldier followed him home and became born to his wife.

In addition to giving the foregoing account and making some other statements, U Tinn Sein, as a child, showed a constellation of what I call "Japanese" traits. One of the most prominent of these was his conspicuous industry. He was indefatigable in working and scorned those who were not. The Burmese are not a lazy people, but their society provided the prototype for the idea that "small is beautiful," and they rarely wish to produce more than they need. When the child Tinn Sein came home from school, he would find his parents sitting at ease and talking amiably together. He would say to them: "Why are you not working? In Tokyo we had to go to work when the siren sounded, and we had to continue until it sounded again."

Another Burmese subject of this group, Maung Sein Win, also claimed to remember the previous life of a Japanese soldier in Upper Burma. He, too, said that he had been killed by a shot from an airplane. He said that he had died near the village where he was born. Unlike U Tinn Sein, he had two birthmarks, a small round one on the front of his left upper chest (*) and a much larger one, also round, on his left upper back (*). The larger one was about 2.5 centimeters in diameter; it was hairless, puckered, and scarlike in appearance. This is the first of eight cases (to be described in this book) with birthmarks corresponding to bullet wounds of entry and exit. The presumed wounds on the Japanese soldier whose life Maung Sein Win remembered were not verified; but I shall later describe cases in which such wounds of entry and exit were verified.

Maung Sein Win exhibited the unusual (for Burma) industriousness of the children who claimed to have been Japanese soldiers. He said that he had been a mechanic in the previous life, and he was gifted in the use of his hands. When he grew up, he built his own house. Perhaps his most unusual behavior was a marked phobia of airplanes. As a child, when he would hear one, he would run toward the nearest house and throw himself under it on the ground. (In Burmese villages, the houses are nearly always elevated off the ground so that there is an open space beneath them.)

Maung Myint Aung was the third Burmese subject of this group who claimed to remember the previous life of a Japanese soldier. He also was born in Upper Burma, in 1972. Unlike U Tinn Sein and Maung Sein Win, however, he said, when he began speaking about a previous life, that he had died in Rangoon, far away from his village. He said that he had been in the Japanese Army that retreated before the British. (As I mentioned, this occurred in the spring of 1945.) He finally found himself, along with four friends, in the Rangoon zoo, where they were in danger of being captured. Preferring death to capture, they all committed suicide. Maung Myint Aung said that he slit his throat, presumably with a large knife or bayonet.

Maung Myint Aung had a prominent birthmark on his neck. It was a horizontal area, about 1 centimeter wide, extending across almost the entire front of his neck. It had slightly increased pigmentation compared with the surrounding skin (Figure 3). It looked much like the healed scar of someone who had slit his throat and survived. I have a photograph of a Virginia man who slit his throat and did not survive (*). It shows a wound closely similar to the one Maung Myint Aung said he gave himself in the life as a Japanese soldier.

To return to Maung Myint Aung's narrative, he said that after dying he remained at the Rangoon zoo until one day he saw his (present) father and followed him home. (Maung Myint Aung's father confirmed that he had gone to the zoo in Rangoon, before Maung Myint Aung's birth. He was completely unaware that any discarnate Japanese soldier had attached himself to him there and followed him 400 kilometers back to his home.) Maung Myint Aung said that his father in Japan had died, but his mother was "still living." (This presumably referred to the time when the Japanese soldier left Japan for service overseas.) He was the oldest of seven children. He was unmarried. He did not give a name for the Japanese soldier, state his rank in the army, or give any address of where he had lived in Japan. He evidently remembered being more prosperous than were his (present) parents, and he sometimes offered to go back to Japan and bring money to them from there. He continued making proposals to go to Japan for money until he was about 7 years old.

Maung Myint Aung was one of many subjects of these cases who showed in their play the vocation of the previous life. He liked to play at being a soldier. He would organize games of soldiers among his playmates, assign himself the role of leader, and say that he was an officer.

In addition, Maung Myint Aung exhibited numerous "Japanese" traits. He preferred sweet foods, as do most Japanese people. He knelt on his knees as Japanese people do, but the Burmese almost never. He worshiped in a style unfamiliar to his parents and showed some resistance to their instructions to him about the forms of worship in Burmese Buddhism. He was hardworking and relatively insensitive to pain and physical discomfort. He was noted to be somewhat harsh and brusque. His father described his behavior as tending to be "crude, like that of a rough and ready soldier." Maung Myint Aung was also troubled by any comments or news adverse to Japan; for example, he did not like to be told that a Japanese soccer team had lost a match.

Lûtfi Sarıkaya, a Turkish boy, had several birthmarks on his chest that showed diminished pigmentation; that is, they were markedly paler than the surrounding skin (*). Lûtfi said that he had been stabbed to death in the previous life. He gave some vague indications of where he had lived in the previous life, but the details were not specific enough to permit solving the case.

Duran İncirgöz (a Turk) was born with a large, round, scarlike birthmark on his right buttock (*). It oozed for some weeks after his birth. When he could speak, he said that he had been shot to death in a brothel. He had a marked phobia of prostitutes and brothels. His case is also unsolved.

Henry Elkin, a Tlingit of Alaska, had a small, roundish, scarlike birthmark on the front of his left chest (*) and a larger, irregularly shaped birthmark, also scarlike, at the same level on his left back (*). These seem to have corresponded to gunshot wounds of entry and exit. Henry Elkin himself, however, had no memories of how the person with whom his parents may have identified him had died.

Maung Aye Kyaw, a subject of Burma, had a large birthmark on the side of his head. It was hairless, puckered, and scarlike (*). He said he remembered the life of a man, Maung Shwe, who had been captured, shot, and killed by Communists at the time of the insurgency in Burma during the early 1950s. Maung Shwe's murderers threw his body into a flooded river, where it floated downstream until it bumped against a dock. From there the owners of the dock pushed it back into the river. One of the owners became Maung Aye Kyaw's mother. She must have become pregnant within a few weeks, perhaps a few days, of the arrival of Maung Shwe's body at her family's dock. As a child, Maung Aye Kyaw remembered being shot and then, in the discarnate state, following Maung Shwe's body as it floated down the river until it came to the dock owned by the family of his mother-to-be. This case illustrates what I call the "geographical factor," which I find helpful in trying to understand why a child of one village has memories of a life in another, often remote village or town, with which the child's family has no obvious connection. Maung Shwe's widow later married and then again became a widow. When Maung Aye Kyaw grew up, he sought out Maung Shwe's widow and married her.

Daw Aye Myint was another subject of Burma, who said that she remembered the previous life of a man who had been struck over the head with a heavy sword or chopping knife. Hers was thus a case of the sex-change type. Her birthmark was a linear area of hairlessness, in part puckered, that extended for 15 centimeters across the top of her head (*). It was oozing at birth and continued to do so for some weeks afterward.

I will now summarize one of the richest cases—as regards details—in this group. It is that of Nirankar Bhatnagar. The previous personality about whom Nirankar talked was clearly identified, but his body was not found, and therefore we have no independent verification of the wound to which Nirankar's birthmark corresponded, as he said it did.

Nirankar was born in Kanpur, Uttar Pradesh, India, in 1935. I did not meet him until 1976, when he was 41 years old. This was, to say the least, a late start in investigating a case. Nevertheless, the case had been investigated in 1938 by S. C. Bose, who wrote a report of it that I have been able to use. In addition, Dr. Satwant Pasricha (who worked with me on the case) and I found that some qualified informants were still living, and their memories seemed sufficiently reliable.

When Nirankar was about 2½ years old, members of his family observed him filling small bottles with water, and when they questioned him about this, he said that his wife was ill and he was going to take medicines to her. He then gave some further details of a previous life—and death during a riot—that he was remembering. He said that his name was Mukhtiar and that Moslems had killed him. One of them—supposedly a friend—had sent for him, but when he arrived at the scene of the riot, he was struck on the head with a baton. He fell down and asked for some water. Instead of being given water, he was stabbed with a dagger.

All these statements did not come out in one flow, but probably over several days. Nirankar's family members were slightly acquainted with the family of a man called Shiv Dayal Mukhtiar whose house was about 100 meters from their own. They knew also that Shiv Dayal had been killed by Moslems during a particularly bloody communal riot that took place in a nearby quarter of Kanpur in March 1931, that is, about 4½ years before Nirankar's birth.

The word *Mukhtiar* is not a personal name, but rather a vocational title given to certain lawyers, of whom Shiv Dayal was one. He had been a much respected, much loved lawyer and municipal leader. The reports of the riot that I studied in the Indian newspapers gave counts of the bodies stacked up in piles, but few names of the killed were published. Shiv Dayal's was one of these. Because of Shiv Dayal's prominence and the slight acquaintance between the families, Nirankar's family knew nearly everything there was to know about how Shiv Dayal had died. That, however, was not much. He had disappeared into the area of the riot, and the police later recovered his body among the corpses. We therefore have no verification of Nirankar's statements that he was struck on the head with a baton and then stabbed.

Nirankar, however, stated one detail about Shiv Dayal's death that was almost certainly not known to members of Nirankar's family and that was correct. They decided to take Nirankar to Shiv Dayal's house, where Shiv Dayal's widow and one of his sons were still living. As they approached the house, Nirankar said:

"My name is inscribed here." In fact, Shiv Dayal's name was written in Urdu on the door. Inside the house, Nirankar met Shiv Dayal's widow and son. He then rebuked the widow for not giving him a gun that he—as Shiv Dayal—had asked for before going into the area of the riot. Shiv Dayal's son (whom we interviewed) had been only 7 years old at the time of his father's death, but he seemed to remember well the events leading up to it. According to him, the man who had sent a message to Shiv Dayal to come to the area of the rioting advised him to bring a gun. His wife, however, somehow got the gun away from Shiv Dayal or, more likely, persuaded him not to go with a firearm, which might have been considered provocative in such an inflamed situation. He left without the gun. This is the detail connected with Shiv Dayal's death that I believe members of Nirankar's family would not have known. Nirankar certainly knew it and said more than once: "If I had been given a gun, I would not have been killed."

To return to Nirankar's first visit to Shiv Dayal's widow, informants credited him with recognizing various objects in the house, such as a typewriter, a walking stick, and shoes that he said were his. He was unable, however, to answer questions that Shiv Dayal's widow put to him about particular documents and debtors.

Shiv Dayal's widow asked Nirankar whether he would like something to eat. Assuming the authoritative air of Indian husbands toward wives (at least of the 1930s), Nirankar replied: "You know what I like." She did, and she sent for rasgoolas, a sweet Indian dessert. Nirankar ate the rasgoolas, drank some water, and asked for betel nut, such as many adult Indians chew as a digestive after meals or between.

As a result of his statements and recognitions (of which I have not given a complete list here), Shiv Dayal's widow fully accepted Nirankar as her husband reborn. She treated him like a husband, sometimes inviting him to lunch and serving him with food that she knew Shiv Dayal had liked. Shiv Dayal's son told us that he was equally convinced that Nirankar was his father reborn.

For his part, Nirankar adopted a paternal attitude toward Shiv Dayal's children. He saved his money to give to them and even sometimes set aside a portion of his food for them. (They were far from needing his assistance; but this was the child's manner of showing affection for them.)

I did not obtain consistent testimony about how long Nirankar continued to remember the previous life. His parents tried to suppress him, but he may have simply stopped speaking about the previous life while he continued to remember it. Eventually, but at what age I do not know, he did forget it.

I mentioned that the first observation of unusual behavior on the part of Nirankar occurred when he was seen filling bottles with water, which he designated as medicine intended for his wife. I am unsure how best to interpret this behavior. Shiv Dayal had been married twice. His first wife, with whom he had several children, died of tuberculosis after a prolonged illness during which Shiv Dayal may well have brought medicines to her, although I did not confirm this conjecture. Shiv Dayal married his second wife only a few months before his death. Subsequently, however, she became ill, and she died in 1938, only a few months after she met Nirankar. She took medicines which her stepchildren sometimes brought to her. Therefore, a second conjecture about Nirankar's behavior with the bottles of water supposes that he had some telepathic awareness that Shiv Dayal's second, still living wife needed medicines. If that is correct, he would be one of several subjects who have shown evidence of paranormal communications with members of the previous personality's family.

Nirankar had no phobias, such as of batons or daggers. Nor did he have a phobia of Moslems. He did, however, have an aversion for them. At times he showed a vengeful attitude toward them, and one informant had heard him say more than once: "That Moslem is coming. I will kill him." At the time I knew Nirankar in the 1970s, he acknowledged still having some dislike of Moslems.

Nirankar's birthmark was a hairless area of increased pigmentation near the top of his head and almost in the midline. It was somewhat irregular in shape, measuring approximately 8 millimeters long and 4 millimeters wide (*). This is one of the few cases for which I did not find a person older than the subject who could assure me that the apparent birthmark had been present at birth. I accept it as a birthmark, however, for two reasons: It did not in any way have the appearance of a scar from a postnatal injury; and although it did have the appearance of a nevus, these are almost never found on the scalp.

Nirankar said that Shiv Dayal had been struck on the head and then stabbed. He was not aware of having had other birthmarks that might have corresponded to a stab wound; and when I examined his chest, I could find none. If we accept Nirankar's account of the sequence of events, Shiv Dayal might have been in a state of obtunded consciousness, or even unconscious, when he was stabbed; and this might explain why Nirankar had only one birthmark. I shall defer further discussion of this possibility until Chapter 14.

5

BIRTHMARKS CORRESPONDING TO WOUNDS VERIFIED BY INFORMANTS' MEMORIES

In this chapter, I present summaries of cases in which informants verified the correspondence between the subject's birthmark or birthmarks and wounds on the previous personality. Such verifications never match in quality what we can obtain from a written record, such as a postmortem report; but, as I shall show later, I believe that we are justified in relying on them in most cases. For all but one of the cases in this chapter, I will condense the report to a single paragraph.

The first case of this group is that of Maung Zaw Thein Lwin, a subject of Burma who remembered the previous life of a man, U Mar Din, who, while trying to rob birds' nests at a temple, had fallen through a weak ceiling board and dropped about 5 meters onto concrete flooring below. He suffered multiple injuries, particularly of the head. Maung Zaw Thein Lwin's birthmark was a large, scarlike area at the back of his head (*). This was at the location of what was probably the most serious of the injuries noted on U Mar Din after he fell onto the concrete floor.

Yvonne Ehrlich was the subject of a same-family case of Brazil. Her case has only meager details and depends on a dream, a single remark she made, some similarities of behavior, and two birthmarks. The birthmarks were areas of distinct redness on the frontal part of her head and at its back. The first of these had faded by the time I examined Yvonne, but the other had persisted (*). Yvonne was identified as the reincarnation of her great-aunt, who had been killed during a bombing raid on Vienna near the end of World War II. Her son confirmed the location of her principal wounds. Yvonne's birthmarks were at the same sites.

Mahmut Ekici was a subject of Turkey who remembered the life of a Turkish partisan engaged in resistance against the French, who were then (the 1920s and 1930s) occupying part of southern Turkey. The partisan was captured and stabbed once, probably with a bayonet, through the liver. Mahmut Ekici had a large depressed birthmark, really a small cavity in the skin, over his liver (*).

Som Pit Hancharoen was a Thai subject who was born with a large oozing birthmark near his left nipple (*). When he could speak, he spoke about the life of a man who, while drunk, had embraced a woman against her wishes. There was a throng at the fair where this occurred. The woman, mingling in the crowd, approached the man from behind, reached around his chest, and plunged a knife into his heart. He had time to say "she stabbed me" before dropping dead. The birthmark might be regarded as an accessory nipple; these sometimes occur in human beings. It also might have had more than one cause.

Ali Uğurlu, the subject of a case in Turkey, was born with multiple birthmarks on his abdomen. They had the appearance of healed stab wounds (*). He remembered the previous life of a man who had got into a fight with another man, who had killed him by stabbing him repeatedly in the abdomen.

The case of this group for which I will present most detail is that of Chanai Choomalaiwong, who was born in central Thailand in 1967. His parents lived separately, and Chanai was at first raised by his mother and maternal grandmother, who owned a duck farm. From the age of 2, he lived alone with his grandmother at a place called Nong La Korn. When Chanai was born, he was found to have two birthmarks, one at the back of his head (Figure 4) and one at the front, above his left eye (Figure 5). At that time his family had no understanding of their possible origin.

When Chanai was about 3 years old, his grandmother noticed that when he played with other children he would pretend that he was a teacher and would also say that he had been a teacher in his last life. Subsequently, he stated further details about this life. He said that he was called Bua Kai and had been shot and killed while on the way to his school. He said that he had parents, a wife, and children. He began to beg his grandmother to take him to Bua Kai's parents and claimed that he could show where they lived at a place called Khao Phra.

Eventually, when Chanai was still less than 4 years old, his grandmother decided to take him to Khao Phra. They went by bus to a town called Khao Sai, which is near Khao Phra. There Chanai led the way to a house. They entered, and Chanai recognized an elderly couple as "his" parents. They were the parents of a schoolteacher called Bua Kai Lawnak, who had been murdered in 1962. They examined Chanai's birthmarks, and these together with his statements impressed them sufficiently so that they invited him to return. On a second visit to Bua Kai's family Chanai recognized other members of the family and also some objects that had belonged to Bua Kai. He answered questions about Bua Kai's possessions with impressive accuracy.

Informants credited Chanai with making 14 correct statements about Bua Kai's life and death; he made one statement that we did not verify. In Chapter 1 I explained why I think most recognitions attributed to the subjects of these cases have little value. Too often, the circumstances permit the possibility, almost the likelihood, that the persons around the subject give him or her cues that could guide the recognitions. Nevertheless, in my report of this case in the monograph I list four recognitions that do not seem vulnerable to this criticism.

The most impressive of these occurred when Chanai was between 5 and 6 years old. He had continued visiting Bua Kai's family, and on this occasion he was with Bua Kai's twin daughters, Tim and Toi. They noticed an old friend of Bua Kai, whom Chanai had never seen before. They called this man over and asked Chanai whether he knew him. Chanai replied: "Yes, his name is San Am." He then went on to say that San Am and he had been friends. This was correct for Bua Kai.

Bua Kai's biography helps us understand Chanai's unusual behavior, and so I will next give an outline of Bua Kai's life. He was born in 1926. He grew up in the area of Khao Sai. He married a girl called Suan, and they had four children, two of whom were the twin daughters already mentioned, Tim and Toi. Suan was pregnant again at the time Bua Kai was killed.

Bua Kai trained and worked as a schoolteacher. That, however, was not his only occupation; he appears to have had a sideline as a gangster. (He had owned two guns.) He also had affairs with other women whose boyfriends or husbands may have objected to these. Someone shot at him while he was attending a fair in Khao Phra, but he escaped serious injury. After this attempted assassination, and perhaps because of it, he applied for a transfer and was assigned to a school near the large town of Tapanhin, which is about 25 kilometers west of Khao Sai.

On the morning of January 23, 1962, Bua Kai left home to go to his school on his bicycle. On the way, he was shot in the head from behind and died almost instantly. The police arrived and took away his body. A doctor examined it and spoke with Suan, who was summoned, and she also saw her husband's body, as did some other persons, including Bua Kai's younger brother Sai. Suan and Sai agreed that the bullet had entered at the back of Bua Kai's head and exited above his left eye. Suan said the doctor had also agreed with this course of the bullet.

Suan had enough knowledge of gunshot wounds to know that a wound of entry is nearly always smaller than the corresponding wound of exit.

By the time I reached the scene of the case in 1979, 17 years had elapsed since Bua Kai's death. No one could remember any longer the name of the doctor who had examined Bua Kai's body. I had the police records searched, and eventually a report of the crime was turned up. It gave the date of the murder, but no other useful information. The police made no arrest in connection with the crime, although this was for lack of evidence, not for lack of suspects. Because there had been no trial, there were no court documents with which a postmortem report would have been filed.

Bua Kai's murder was widely known in the region where he lived. My inquiries showed that some members of the two families concerned had had some acquaintance, but there had been no social relationships between them. Chanai's grandmother had no idea where she would find herself when Chanai finally persuaded her to take him to Khao Sai; she clearly did not know where Bua Kai's family lived.

Chanai belonged to a small group of subjects who preserved memories past the age of 7 or 8. He was also one of the few to say that he saw the previous personality's body after its death. In 1979, at the age of 11, he made the following statement:

> I don't know who shot me, because he shot me from the back. I was not conscious when I died. Afterward though, I felt my soul leaving the body. I could see myself lying on the road. My legs were still twitching. My blood was running onto the road.

Despite Chanai's just cited denial that he knew who had killed Bua Kai, on another occasion he said that he did know who the murderer was and expressed anger as he said this. In this he joined many other subjects who have shown anger toward the killer of the person whose life they remember.

Among other unusual behavior, I have already mentioned Chanai's play at teaching. He was also interested in guns and spoke about a wish to be a policeman or a soldier when he grew up; he did not intend to be a schoolteacher.

Chanai showed in several matters what I call an "adult attitude." By this expression I mean behavior toward other persons that an older person would ordinarily show toward younger persons, and sometimes toward persons of the previous personality's own age; it is often accompanied by a sense of superiority toward other persons. For example, Chanai expected Bua Kai's twin daughters to address him as "Father." Because they were 17 years old when he was 3, they objected; but he said that if they did not call him "Father," he would not speak to them, and they capitulated. Sai, Bua Kai's younger brother, would not show Chanai the deference due an older brother, and Chanai tended to shun him when he was in Sai's area. Chanai also showed a proprietary attitude toward Bua Kai's possessions. He became annoyed when he learned that some of them had been modified after Bua Kai's death.

For some years, Chanai came to visit Bua Kai's family in Khao Sai and Khao Phra. Sometimes he went with his grandmother, but he also visited them covertly by himself, on the bus; his grandmother would then have to come after him and bring him home. When he visited Tim and Toi, he brought them pieces of sugar cane, which Bua Kai had frequently done.

For their part, Bua Kai's family, after some initial surprise and skepticism, came to accept Chanai fully as Bua Kai reborn. There was even talk of their adopting him, but his grandmother would not allow this.

Figure 4 shows the small round birthmark at the back of Chanai's head. It was about 0.5 centimeter in diameter, hairless, puckered, and with increased pigmentation. This birthmark corresponded to the wound of entry on Bua Kai. Figure 5 shows a larger birthmark at the front of Chanai's head. It was irregular in shape and measured about 2 centimeters long and 0.5 centimeter wide. It also was scarlike, hairless, and had increased pigmentation. It corresponded to the bullet wound of exit on Bua Kai.

I was able to meet Chanai again in 1986. He was then 18, married, and working as a telephone lineman. He said that he still remembered some details of the previous life, but had forgotten others. I examined Chanai's birthmarks again, and a colleague arranged for them to be photographed for me. The birthmark near Chanai's forehead had changed little since 1979 (*), but the one at the back of the head had moved up in relation to surrounding anatomical sites (*).

Maung Tin Win, a subject of Burma, remembered the previous life of a bandit (called *dacoit* in Burma, as in India) who was betrayed to government soldiers and shot. Maung Tin Win had a small round birthmark in his right lower abdomen (*) and a much larger birthmark on his right back (*). These corresponded to bullet wounds of entry and exit on the bandit whose life he remembered. Maung Tin Win is the fourth subject I have so far described with two birthmarks corresponding to gunshot wounds of entry and exit. In Chapter 12 I discuss the importance of these cases.

Yahya Balcı, a Turkish subject, remembered the life of a man who became involved in a quarrel with another man. His adversary shot and killed him. Yahya Balcı had a small, almost perfectly round birthmark on his left abdomen (*). There was some question about his also having a birthmark on his back, presumably corresponding to the wound of exit, but when I examined him carefully I could not convince myself that he had such a mark. If one had been there, it had faded.

Aristide Kolotey, a Ghanian, was born with a long linear birthmark that extended almost from his neck down the front of his chest and to his lower abdomen (*). It showed diminished pigmentation. Aristide was said to be the reincarnation of an uncle who had gone swimming and drowned. The uncle's body was washed up on the shore and found to have a "cut in the middle of the chest." It was supposed that the uncle had dived onto rocks that he did not see and cut himself as he hit them. Aristide had no imaged memories of the uncle's life or death; but he did have a marked phobia of water.

The last subject of this chapter was Daw Aye Than, who was born with a long, scarlike birthmark extending across her right upper abdomen onto the left lower chest between her breasts (*). She remembered the life of a young girl who was caught in a fire from which she could not escape. The intense heat of the fire had expanded the air in the girl's intestines until they and the abdominal wall burst. Daw Aye Than's birthmark was said to correspond to the place where the girl's abdomen had broken open. Daw Aye Than also had asymmetrical breasts; her right breast was markedly lower than her left one (*). Daw Aye Than believed that the asymmetry of her breasts derived from the previous life; and it is conjecturable that the injured area of the body of the child whose life she remembered was larger than the visible linear birthmark suggested.

6

BIRTHMARKS CORRESPONDING TO WOUNDS VERIFIED BY MEDICAL RECORDS

The cases that I describe in this chapter belong to the most important group in the entire collection. The medical records, usually postmortem reports, verify the correspondence between the birthmarks and the wounds with a certitude sometimes approached but never reached by the testimonies of informants drawing on their memories.

I will present two of the twelve cases in some detail and give shorter summaries of the remaining ones.

Metin Köybaşı was born in the village of Hatun Köy, near İskenderun, Turkey, on June 11, 1963. Even before his birth, he had been provisionally identified, on the basis of dreams his parents had had, as the reincarnation of a relative (Haşim Köybaşı), who had been killed some 5 months before, during a postelection riot in the village.

At his birth Metin was found to have a birthmark on the right side of the front of his neck. It was a small area of increased pigmentation (*). No informant told me to what wound this birthmark corresponded, and I did not know until I examined the postmortem report on Haşim Köybaşı. This showed that the bullet which killed Haşim had entered his head behind the left ear and almost exited on the right side of the front of the neck. It did not, however, fully penetrate the skin; as sometimes happens, the resistance of the skin stopped the bullet before it exited. The pathologist had made a small incision and extracted the bullet. The birthmark therefore corresponded to the pathologist's postmortem wound. As for the bullet wound of entry, I could see nothing distinctly corresponding to that behind Metin's left ear. Nevertheless, I photographed the area and on the developed photograph found a round area of increased pigmentation (*). I believe that this corresponded to the wound of entry. (Perhaps I had failed to see the mark because of insufficient light when I examined Metin looking for it.)

Like many other children of these cases Metin showed powerful attitudes of vengefulness toward the man who had shot Haşim. He once tried to take his father's gun and shoot this person, but was fortunately restrained. He later became more pacific.

Tali Sowaid was born in August 1965 in the tiny village of Btebyat in the mountains east of Beirut, Lebanon. He had circular birthmarks of increased pigmentation on each cheek. They were not prominent and yet, once seen, were easily discernible (*).

Soon after Tali began to speak, he started referring to the life of a man who had lived in the village of Btechney (which is about 4 kilometers from Btebyat at the top of its valley). He described how he had been having a cup of coffee before leaving for work when a man came up to him and shot him.

What Tali was saying corresponded exactly to the murder of a man called Said Abul-Hisn, who lived at Btechney. The assailant, a person of noted mental instability, seems to have mistaken Said for another man against whom he had a grudge. He came up to Said stealthily and shot him at close range. The bullet entered one side of Said's face and exited at the other, traversing the tongue on the way. Said was taken to a hospital in Beirut and given emergency surgical treatment. His tongue having swollen, it was necessary to make a hole in his windpipe (tracheostomy) in order to provide an adequate airway. Somehow, Said fell out of bed, and when this happened, his tracheostomy tube must have become obstructed, and he died. The incident of falling out of bed just before dying figured in Tali's memories.

I was able to study the hospital record in this case. It showed that the birthmark on Tali's left cheek, which was the smaller of the two, corresponded to the wound of entry, and the larger birthmark on the right cheek corresponded to the wound of exit. (This is the sixth case that I have so far described with birthmarks corresponding to bullet wounds of entry and exit.)

Tali's family owned their modest house, but his father was poor. In contrast, Said had been prosperous, and his elegant house contrasted markedly with the humble dwelling of Tali's family. Tali sometimes made invidious comparisons about the differences in the economic statuses of the two families. He identified strongly with Said and asked his family to call him "Said."

Tali showed a difficulty in articulating properly. He had special trouble in pronouncing certain "s" sounds, which require elevating the tongue. I interpret this defect as a possible residue of the damage to Said's tongue when the bullet passed through it.

Alan Gamble, a Tsimshian, was born in Hartley Bay, British Columbia, Canada, on February 5, 1945. On the basis of a dream and two birthmarks, he was identified as the reincarnation of Walter Wilson, a near relative, who had died several years before Alan's birth under the following circumstances.

Walter Wilson accompanied a friend, who owned a seine boat, when he went fishing off the coast of British Columbia. They were cruising near the shore when Walter noticed a mink running along near the water, and he decided to have a shot at it. The seine boat was towing a skiff, and Walter's shotgun was in the skiff with the barrel pointing toward the bow. He picked it up by the muzzle, but it slipped, the butt hit a board, and the gun discharged. The shots entered Walter's left hand, where he had just grasped the gun, and exited at his wrist. He bled profusely. His friend applied a crude tourniquet and turned the boat toward Prince Rupert, the closest town with a hospital. He was not, however, trained in first aid, and Prince Rupert was 10 hours away. The friend did not know to release the tourniquet from time to time, and when they finally arrived at Prince Rupert, Walter was unconscious and already suffering from incipient gangrene of the arm. Antibiotics were not available then and there. In the hospital, doctors amputated Walter's hand and part of his forearm, but this did not save his life, and he died in the hospital on February 18, 1942.

Walter's friend, the owner of the seine boat, was grief-stricken over Walter's death. Some uninformed and unkind gossips magnified the friend's suffering when they began to hint that he was responsible for Walter's death. He was therefore greatly moved when Alan, as he began to speak, talked about Walter's accidental death in a way that fully exonerated Walter's friend.

Otherwise, Alan made few statements about Walter's life. On one occasion, when Alan was still a young child, he reacted fearfully when he saw a shotgun shell. He did not, however, develop a phobia of guns, and in adulthood he hunted with a gun.

Alan's two birthmarks were on his left hand and wrist. The smaller one (barely visible) was on the palm of the hand (*), and it corresponded to the gunshot wound of entry on Walter. The larger birthmark, which was much more prominent, was on the back of the wrist (*), and it corresponded to the gunshot wound of exit on Walter.

Sunita Singh was born in the Mainpuri District of Uttar Pradesh, India, in August 1967. At birth she was found to have an extremely large birthmark of the port-wine stain type. It extended over her upper right chest (*) and much of her right arm (*). In addition, she had three birthmarks on the lower part of the right side of her neck and the upper part of her chest (*).

Sunita's family did not understand her birthmarks until she was a few years old and began to speak about a previous life. Her grandmother happened to take her on a social visit to a neighboring village, where Sunita noticed a man and said: "He is my son." She gave the man's name, Ranvir. One of the women in this village seemed to frighten and even terrify her. After this, Sunita stated details of how in a previous life she had lived in this particular village. She had been murdered there, she said, by her daughter-in-law.

Sunita's statements referred to the life of a woman called Ram Dulari, who had lived with her son and daughter-in-law in the village where Sunita had become frightened. Her son, Ranvir, was often away, and the daughter-in-law had affairs with other men during his absence. Ram Dulari came to know of these and openly expressed her disapproval. In revenge, the daughter-in-law hired professional killers, who broke into the house at night (simulating a burglary) and killed Ram Dulari with a sword. Although the police made no arrests after Ram Dulari's murder, information and conjectures about it diffused into the surrounding villages, including Sunita's. Sunita's father thus knew normally everything that she stated about the previous life. Her mother, however, came from another village and said that she knew nothing about Ram Dulari's murder until Sunita began speaking about it. No one could imagine that Sunita's parents would have encouraged her to identify with Ram Dulari.

Sunita showed a marked fear of Ram Dulari's daughter-in-law when she happened to see her. It was the sight of this woman that had frightened her when she first went to Ram Dulari's village. On another occasion of seeing this woman, Sunita, cowering with fear, told her grandmother: "She will kill me again."

The postmortem report that we obtained showed a satisfactory correspondence between the sword wounds on Ram Dulari's neck and chest and Sunita's birthmarks. We learned that Ram Dulari's body was not washed before it was cremated. I believe the port-wine stain birthmarks on Sunita's chest and arm corresponded to the blood left on Ram Dulari's body when it was cremated.

Nasruddin Shah was born in a village of the Shahjahanpur District of Uttar Pradesh, India, in April 1962. His family were Moslems. His father was a poor, landless laborer. Nasruddin was born with several birthmarks, of which the most prominent was a lens-shaped birthmark on his left chest (*). His family did not understand its significance until Nasruddin began to speak about a previous life.

When he did speak, he said that he was a Thakur, that is, a member of the second highest ranking caste of Hindus. Without saying so explicitly, he indicated that he came from a nearby village called Phargana. He said that he was called Hardev Baksh Singh and had been killed with a spear during a quarrel over cattle. These and other statements that Nasruddin made were correct for the life of a man called Hardev Baksh Singh, a Thakur landowner of Phargana. During a quarrel over cattle, which became violent, one of his adversaries drove a spear through his left upper chest, and he died almost immediately. The postmortem report confirmed the close correspondence in location between Nasruddin's birthmark when he was born and the fatal spear wound in Hardev Baksh Singh. By the time we first met and examined Nasruddin (when he was 13 years old), the birthmark had migrated to a position lower on his chest than the position it had formerly occupied. (In Chapter 11 I discuss the movement of some birthmarks relative to other anatomical features.) A birthmark on Nasruddin's head had faded by this time.

The most remarkable feature of this case—apart from the principal birthmark—was Nasruddin's "Thakur behavior." Although born a Moslem, he considered himself a Hindu; moreover, he regarded himself as one of particular distinction. For example, he refused to engage in activities, such as collecting cow dung for fuel, that most village boys in India would undertake without question. Nasruddin also resisted the Islamic religion; he would not say Islamic prayers or go to the mosque.

Nasruddin's parents knew that reincarnation is not part of the teaching of their religion, but Nasruddin's statements and behavior convinced them that he was the reincarnation of Hardev Baksh Singh.

Henry Demmert III, a Tlingit, was born in Juneau, Alaska, on October 5, 1968. His parents separated soon after his birth, and he was raised (and adopted) by his grandfather, Henry Demmert, Sr., and his second wife, Gertrude.

Shortly before Henry's birth, Gertrude Demmert dreamed that her husband's deceased son by his first wife, Henry Demmert, Jr., was looking for his father and her. (In the dream he was *not* looking for the couple who became Henry's parents, but, as it turned out, for those who adopted and raised Henry Demmert III.)

When Henry Demmert III was born, he was found to have a birthmark on his upper left chest in the region of the heart (*). On the basis of Gertrude's dream and this birthmark, Henry was identified as the reincarnation of Henry Demmert, Jr. and given the latter's Tlingit name.

The life of Henry Demmert, Jr. was brief and tragic. He was born in Juneau in 1929. I think his mother must have died when he was still an infant, and he was raised by his father and his father's second wife, who was Gertrude Demmert. When he grew up, he spent some time in the Armed Forces and then became a fisherman. He married and had two children. He was a heavy drinker of alcohol.

On March 6, 1957, he attended a party that lasted all night and where alcohol was abundantly consumed. Around 5:00 a.m. of the following morning he was stabbed in the heart. He was rushed to a hospital, but died less than 2 hours after being wounded. I was able to obtain a copy of the death certificate for Henry Demmert, Jr. It recorded his death as due to an "accidental self-inflicted wound." Some further details included: "Laceration of the left lung and heart causing exsanguination....knife wound pierced the heart."

Henry Demmert, Jr.'s family regarded his death as a case of murder. The police, however, found no witnesses willing to charge a suspect, and they made no arrests. It is possible that in struggling with another man, who may also have had a knife, Henry Demmert Jr.'s knife became pushed into his chest with the fatal consequences described.

Henry Demmert III's birthmark was located below and to the side of his left nipple. It was an elongated area of increased pigmentation, about 3 centimeters long and 8 millimeters wide. It was slightly narrower toward the inside, so that its shape was roughly that of the profile of a single-edged knife (*).

Henry Demmert III belongs to the small group of subjects, who, although identified as being someone reincarnated, say little or nothing about the presumed previous life. When he was about 2 years old, he made the only two statements he ever uttered about the previous life. He said, pointing to his birthmark, that he had "got hurt there." He added that this had happened when he "was big."

Unlike some other subjects who have remembered the previous life of an alcoholic or heavy drinker of alcohol, Henry Demmert III, when he was young, showed no desire for alcohol.

Narong Yensiri was born in the village of Tung Yai in northern Thailand on October 4, 1976. At his birth, his parents noticed several prominent birthmarks, of which the largest was at the lower part of his chest near the midline (*). Large parts of the skin of his back were heavily pigmented (*).

When Narong became able to speak, he began to refer to the life of his maternal grandfather. The grandfather was called Pan Srisukit, and he had been murdered under mysterious circumstances 2 years before Narong's birth.

Pan Srisukit was a farmer who also engaged in cattle trading and perhaps in stealing cattle. One day, two men came to visit him. They ate and drank together, and then Pan Srisukit went off with them without telling his wife where he was going or when he would return. Although somewhat accustomed to such behavior on the part of her husband, Pan Srisukit's wife became concerned when he did not return home after a couple of days. She notified the police, and a search eventually led to the discovery of Pan Srisukit's body in the forest. A doctor was called, and he examined the body at the scene. His report, which I could study, showed a good correspondence between wounds on the body and the birthmarks on Narong.

Pan Srisukit's wife had his body cremated at the site where it was found. The increased pigmentation on Narong's trunk may have corresponded to blood left on Pan Srisukit's body when it was cremated.

Necip Ünlütaşkıran was born in Adana, Turkey, in 1951. Necip's mother had a dream before he was born in which a man she did not recognize showed himself to her with bleeding wounds. She did not know how to interpret this dream, but it made some sense when she saw, after Necip's birth, that he had seven birthmarks. Some of these were more prominent than others, and a few had faded by the time I first examined Necip, when he was about 13 years old (*).

Necip was late in speaking and late also, compared with other subjects of these cases, in speaking about a previous life. From the age of 6 on he began to say that he had children and asked his mother to take him to them. He said that he had lived in Mersin (a city about 80 kilometers from Adana). He said that his name was Necip and that he had been stabbed; as he described the stabbing, he pointed to various parts of his body to indicate where he had been stabbed.

His parents at first paid little attention to his statements, which they found more annoying than interesting. Their stance changed when Necip was about 12 years old. His mother took him to meet her father, who was then living, with his second wife, in a village near Mersin. Necip had never met his grandfather's second wife before, but he suddenly said that he recognized her as from the previous life that he claimed to have lived in Mersin. She had known a man in Mersin called Necip Budak, and she was able to confirm the accuracy of Necip's statements. This meeting increased Necip's wish to go to Mersin, and his grandfather took him there. There he recognized several members of the family of Necip Budak. They further confirmed the accuracy of Necip's statements for the life of Necip Budak.

It seems that Necip Budak had been a quarrelsome sort of person, especially when drunk. One day he began teasing and then taunting an acquaintance, who, perhaps drunk himself, stabbed Necip Budak repeatedly with a knife. Necip Budak collapsed on the street and was taken to a hospital, where his wounds were noted and where he died the next day.

Among the statements Necip made, the most impressive was his claim that he had once stabbed "his" (Necip Budak's) wife in the leg and that she thereafter had a scar on her leg. Necip Budak's widow admitted the truth of this statement, and, taking some ladies into a back room, she showed them the scar on her thigh.

Necip expressed great affection toward the children of Necip Budak and fond attachment toward his wife. Indeed, he manifested keen jealousy regarding her second husband and wanted to tear up a photograph of this man.

In the number of wounds matching birthmarks—six in all—Necip's case exceeds all other cases (having medical documents) that I have investigated. In the monograph I give a tabular summary of these and show their correspondence to the wounds on Necip Budak recorded in the hospital where he died.

Hanumant Saxena was born in 1955 in the Farrukhabad District of the state of Uttar Pradesh, India. Not long before Hanumant's mother conceived him, she dreamed that a man of the same village called Maha Ram appeared to her. Maha Ram had been shot dead only a few weeks earlier. In the dream, Maha Ram said to Hanumant's mother: "I am coming to you." Having said that, he lay down on a cot. The dream ended there.

When Hanumant was born, his parents noticed a large birthmark on the lower part of his chest near the midline (Figure 6). It was irregular in shape and really consisted of several birthmarks close together. The birthmark had diminished pigmentation in comparison with the surrounding skin. Hanumant later said that as a young child he had had no pain in the area of the birthmark, but his parents said that he sometimes had complained of pain there. He himself said that intermittently from the age of about 14 on he had had some pain in the area of the birthmark.

Hanumant's birthmark corresponded closely in location to the fatal wound on Maha Ram, and I shall say a little about him and how he died. Maha Ram was born in about 1905 in the same village as Hanumant, and his house was not more than 250 meters from that of Hanumant's family. He was a farmer who had some land and owned a bullock-cart, which he sometimes drove for hire. He married and had five children. His younger brother described him as a "simple, good fellow." He had no known enemies. Nevertheless, on the evening of September 28, 1954, he was standing near a teashop at the crossroads, not far from his home, when someone shot him at close range with a shotgun. He died almost immediately. His assailant fled, and because he had not been identified, the police made no arrests. Because Maha Ram was such a harmless person, he might have been killed accidentally, his murderer, in the dark, having mistaken him for someone else.

The postmortem report showed that the main charge of pellets had hit Maha Ram in the lower chest in the midline; there was some scattering of wounds from shot around the principal wound. The Indian doctor who examined the postmortem report with me (and who had no knowledge of the location of Hanumant's birthmark) sketched in the location of wounds on a human figure drawing (Figure 7). This shows the almost exact correspondence between the wounds and Hanumant's birthmark.

Hanumant began to speak when he was about 1 year old. When he was about 3 years old, he started referring to the life of Maha Ram. He said that he was Maha Ram, and, pointing to his birthmark, he said that he had been shot there. He made a few other statements that were correct for Maha Ram, and he recognized some people and places familiar to Maha Ram. In particular, he recognized Maha Ram's bullocks, which was perhaps not difficult because the bullocks were standing outside Maha Ram's house.

Hanumant liked to visit Maha Ram's house and to be with Maha Ram's mother, who still lived there. Hanumant's mother told us that he talked about the previous life until he was 5 or 6 years old, but his father said that he continued to visit Maha Ram's house until the age of 10. Unlike many other subjects of these cases, however, Hanumant never seems to have become intensely involved with the memories of the previous life.

Although I first learned of this case in 1964, it was in what was then for me a particularly remote part of Uttar Pradesh, and I did not reach the scene of the case until 1971. By this time Hanumant was already 16 years old, but the informants seemed to have a good recollection of the main events in the development of the case. Two of them did not support Hanumant's claim to be Maha Ram reborn. Maha Ram's wife declined to be interviewed, possibly because she mistook us for some kind of government officials whom it was better to avoid; and Maha Ram's oldest son rejected the claim, apparently because Hanumant had not recognized him. The other major informants endorsed Hanumant's statement that he was Maha Ram reborn.

Before leaving this case, I will draw attention to the possibility that there are many like it in India that neither our team nor anyone else ever learns about, let alone investigates. This case received no outside publicity, and we came across it almost accidentally. A systematic search for such cases in its area would undoubtedly reveal many others like it. Indeed, a judge of this district advised me to drop all my other projects and move to Farrukhabad. The homicide rate was extremely high there, and the judge seemed aware of the connection between violent death and cases of children who claim to remember previous lives.

Sunita Khandelwal was born in the town of Laxmangarh in the state of Rajasthan, India, on September 19, 1969. Sunita's father, Radhey Shyam Khandelwal, was a dealer in grains, seeds, and fertilizers. Despite owning his own business, he lived in modest circumstances, and I judged him to be a member of the lower middle classes.

Immediately after Sunita's birth, she was noticed to have a large birthmark on the right side of her head. When Sunita was born, the birthmark was bleeding, but her family applied talcum powder to it, and the bleeding stopped after 3 days. The mark was an approximately round, hairless, heavily pigmented area. It was slightly elevated above the surrounding skin and slightly puckered. When Sunita was 9½ years old, the birthmark was about 2.5 centimeters in diameter (*). At her birth, Sunita was not identified as being the reincarnation of anyone in particular, and her family offered themselves no interpretation of her birthmark.

An interpretation came when Sunita, at the age of about 2, first began to refer to a previous life. She said that she was from Kota, where she said she had parents and two brothers. She added further details, such as that her family had a silver shop and a safe. At about the same time or a little later, Sunita said that she had fallen down "from a small height." She pointed to the area of the birthmark on her head and said: "Look here. I have fallen."

Laxmangarh is a small town with about 5,000 inhabitants. Kota, in contrast, is one of the largest cities in Rajasthan and in 1971 had a population of about 300,000. Rajasthan is the largest state in India, and, although both communities are in it, they are 360 kilometers apart.

What Sunita was saying about a life in Kota made no sense to Sunita's family. They had never been to Kota and had no connections with it. Nevertheless, Sunita asked and then demanded to be taken there. She had, however, given no personal names, and even when she added the details that her cousin (in the previous life) had pushed her down (before her fall) and that she had been 8 years old, her family had no substantial clues for finding in Kota the family to which she was referring.

Eventually, when Sunita was 5, a friend of the family urged Sunita's parents to allow her to be taken to Kota with the thought that perhaps a family corresponding to her statements could after all be found. The discovery of such a family might, it was hoped, please and appease Sunita, who had, from time to time, been refusing to eat unless she was taken to Kota. By the time Sunita was taken to Kota, she had stated a few more details, such as the quarter (Chauth Mata Bazaar) where the (previous) family's silver shop was located. She had also stated that the family's caste was that of the Banias (the businessman's caste), although this added little new information, because silversmiths would almost inevitably be Banias. Having arrived at Kota, the group set out to enquire among the silversmiths of Chauth Mata Bazaar for any family who had lost a daughter from falling.

They thus came to the shop of Prabhu Dayal Maheshwari. He had had a daughter, Sakuntala, who had fallen from a balcony and died soon afterward. She had been 8 years old. Sakuntala had been playing with her cousin on a balcony that had an extremely low railing. They might have been pushing each other playfully. Somehow Sakuntala lost her balance, went over the railing, and landed head first on the concrete floor below. Her mother rushed to her and found her unconscious with blood running out of one ear. She summoned her husband, who immediately took Sakuntala to the hospital, where she died a few hours later, on April 28, 1968. The hospital records showed that when she was admitted she was still unconscious and bleeding from the right ear. At that time Kota had no neurosurgeon, and treatment was entirely palliative. The hospital record gave a provisional diagnosis of "head injury." The bleeding from the ear indicated a fracture of the base of the skull. Death would have been due to hemorrhage and swelling of the brain.

As I mentioned, Sunita had not given any personal names, and so the question arose of whether some other family of Kota who had lost a daughter from falling might have matched Sunita's statements as well as that of Prabhu Dayal Maheshwari. This led me first to initiate a search through the medical records of the hospital in Kota where Sakuntala had died, which was the hospital to which all serious cases of head injuries would be taken. The records showed that only three other females (besides Sakuntala) had died of head injuries during 1968. The ages of these females were not given, and they might have been children or older women; nor were the causes of their injuries given, so they might have been injured in falls, in vehicular accidents, or otherwise. Still, there were other years to consider, and if one allowed for a period of 5 years before 1968, as many as a dozen girls might have died of head injuries in Kota during the 5 years before and including 1968.

The next step was to appraise the likelihood that all the other details stated by Sunita could apply as well to some other family. Before she went to Kota, Sunita had made 25 statements of which 21 were correct for Sakuntala, 2 incorrect and 2 unverified. In Kota she made 4 more statements, 3 correct and 1 unverified. Individually, many of her statements were nonspecific and would have applied equally to other families. Taken collectively, however, I think they would not.

A final point of importance is that the visit of Sunita to Kota became well known, and her case generated considerable publicity when her statements led to the family of Sakuntala. A Kota newspaper published an account of the case within a few days of Sunita's first visit. None of this public awareness brought forth information about another candidate family with the suggestion that it matched Sunita's statements as well as or better than Sakuntala's. After a careful appraisal of all the facts, I became convinced that Sakuntala was the correct child and that she alone had had a life and death with details that matched Sunita's statements.

I said that Sunita's parents had never been to Kota before the case developed. Prabhu Dayal had never been to Laxmangarh and did not, at the time the case developed, even know where it was located. Our enquiries did not end there, however; continuing them, we learned that Sunita's maternal uncle, who lived in Jaipur (the capital of Rajasthan), was also a silversmith and that he had been to Kota and had even had some business dealings with Prabhu Dayal. He had not, however, had any social relationships with him and knew nothing about the death of Prabhu Dayal's daughter. I concluded that he could not have been the conduit for Sunita's information about Sakuntala's family in Kota.

In most of these cases, the two families concerned exchange one or several visits, and they may keep up such exchanges for a few years, but rarely for longer. Eventually, they seem to go their own ways and resume lives independent of each other. This case presented an exception. Dr. Satwant Pasricha, who had initiated our investigation of the case in the 1970s, continued to follow it until 1990. Sunita had long since forgotten the details of the previous life, but she had maintained an affectionate relationship with Sakuntala's family and continued to visit them, especially on festive occasions. When, in 1989, Sunita married a law student, Sakuntala's family contributed generously to the costs of the wedding, just as if she were their own daughter.

Dellâl Beyaz was born in Samandağ, Turkey, in July 1970. At her birth she was found to have a substantial birthmark at the top of her head, and it oozed for some days after her birth.

As have some other subjects of these cases, Dellâl gave the first indications of having memories of a previous life when her mother overheard her talking to herself. She seemed to be calling to someone for help. Gradually she communicated details about the life of a woman who, hanging out clothes to dry on the roof of a house, stepped back, and fell through a hole in the roof. She said that she was from Kavaslı. This is a district of the village of Odabaşı, which adjoins Antakya, the capital city of the province of Hatay; it is about 30 kilometers from Samandağ.

Dellâl's statements would have gone unverified longer than they did if a man from Odabaşı who had relatives in Samandağ had not happened to hear about them when he came to Samandağ on a visit. Dellâl's statements seemed to fit closely the life and death of a woman called Zehide Köse, who had lived and died at Odabaşı.

Zehide had been doing just what Dellâl had said. She had been on the roof of a new house hanging out clothes to dry. A stairway opened on the roof without any guarding rail around the opening. Without realizing that the opening was there, Zehide had stepped back and, losing her balance, had fallen into the hole of the stairway. She hit the concrete below, head first. Taken to a hospital, she died there the following day of injuries to her skull and brain.

The hospital record, which I examined, confirmed the cause of Zehide's death. It made no mention of any damage to the scalp that would have corresponded to the birthmark at the top of Dellâl's head; but this could easily have been overlooked beneath Zehide's hair.

I first examined Dellâl's birthmark when she was a little over 5 years old. It was a round, hairless area almost at the center of the top of her head. It was a little less than 1 centimeter in diameter. It resembled the scar of a healed wound (*).

Dellâl was one of the few Turkish subjects to describe an event that occurred after death in the previous life. She gave a correct description of the location of Zehide's grave.

Wilfred Meares, a Haida, was born in Queen Charlotte City, British Columbia, Canada, on November 22, 1961. Before she conceived him, Wilfred's mother, Ruby Meares, had had two dreams about a deceased relative, Victor Smart, who, she said, "kept coming to me." Even before that, this same relative, while he was still living, had said that, if he were to reincarnate, he would like to return as Ruby Meares's child.

Victor Smart was an amiable person, but he was an alcoholic. He also had the dangerous habit of riding in the passenger seat of a car with his back to the door. One day he was being driven with some friends in a car and was sitting in this fashion when the car crashed. The door opened, Victor shot out, and his head hit the pavement. The force was great enough so that he bit his tongue and broke his neck, dying instantly. I obtained a copy of the report of his death at the hospital to which his body was taken; it contained the details I have just given.

Wilfred's birthmark was a hairless area at the back of his head that, when he was 12 years old, measured about 2 centimeters long and 5 millimeters wide (*).

When Wilfred could speak, he made a few statements about the life of Victor Smart. He showed friendships and animosities toward members of the family that accorded with those of Victor Smart.

Wilfred had a precocious interest in alcohol and would hang around adults who were drinking, expecting them to serve him some alcohol. It was observed, however, that he was always polite about this matter and never took a drink without being offered and given one. Ruby Meares told me that Victor Smart also had this admirable trait.

7

BIRTHMARKS CORRESPONDING TO SURGICAL WOUNDS AND OTHER SKIN LESIONS ON DECEASED PERSONS

The deceased persons (or, as I call them, the previous personalities) involved in the 31 cases that I described in the last three chapters all died violently. (We know this for the verified cases and may permissibly assume it for the five unverified cases of Chapter 4.) In this chapter I describe eight cases in which the death was natural. To be sure, in four of these cases death followed a surgical operation, and I suppose surgery is a kind of violence; still, it is one to which the parties involved ordinarily consent, and I believe I am warranted in counting deaths that follow surgery as natural.

The first case of the group has few data: a dream, a birthmark, and some behavior appropriate for the woman of whom Susan Wilson, the subject, was the supposed reincarnation. By its size and position, however, the birthmark seems significant in the identification of the person, Susan Ford, as the correct previous personality.

Susan Ford, a Tlingit, was born in Juneau, Alaska, on September 30, 1910. Her mother died soon after her birth, and she was raised by her father and step-mother, Walter and Rosemary Ford. Susan Ford's mother and Susan Wilson's were cousins, as were their fathers. When Susan Ford was just over 24 years old, she became ill with what her death certificate described as "lobular pneumonia." She had had pleurisy and a surgical drainage of her chest, presumably to drain off an empyema or pleural fluid. She died within a few days, at most, of the pleural drainage, on November 2, 1934.

Susan Wilson was born some 6 years later, on September 5, 1940. Before her birth someone—I did not learn who—had a dream connecting the baby that was about to be born with Susan Ford. When, after Susan's birth, her large birthmark was noticed, she was identified as the reincarnation of Susan Ford and given her name.

The birthmark was a large heavily pigmented nevus. It was located on the left side of the chest at the lower margin of the left breast. It was irregularly rectangular in shape, and during Susan's adulthood it measured about 3 centimeters by 2 centimeters (*). Susan told me that the birthmark had been farther toward her back when she was younger than it later became. It had migrated forward as she grew. The birthmark was at a site where a pleural effusion or empyema secondary to pneumonia might be surgically drained.

When Susan became able to speak, she somehow drew attention to the birthmark on her chest; later, however, her mother could not remember what she had said about it.

Susan showed an unusual attachment to Susan Ford's family. She greatly enjoyed seeing them and would take them a portion of whatever food she cooked for herself. In some other respects, such as in a love of music and a tendency to be unusually active, she was said to resemble Susan Ford.

Muhittin Yılmaz was born at Yenice, near Tarsus, in Turkey, in 1960. Soon after his birth, his mother noticed that he had a red horizontal birthmark in the right upper quadrant of his abdomen. The birthmark subsequently faded somewhat, but was still visible and easily photographed when Muhittin was 15 years old (*). On the basis of this birthmark and of two dreams had by members of the family, Muhittin was judged to be the reincarnation of his paternal grandfather, Muhittin Uğur Yılmaz.

Muhittin Uğur Yılmaz was a farmer who also owned and operated a café in Yenice. He drank alcohol excessively and continued to do so up to the time of his death. In the 1950s he developed a disease of some internal organ and underwent a surgical operation. I did not learn the nature of his illness, but jaundice was one of its symptoms, and his widow said that he had died of cancer. (I was unable to obtain a medical record for this case.) Muhittin's birthmark corresponded closely to a transverse surgical incision that would be made in the hope, among other possibilities, of removing an obstructive gallstone or perhaps a cancer of the head of the pancreas.

This being a same-family case, no one would have expected Muhittin to make statements outside normal knowledge in the family. He was, however, credited with some unusual statements and recognitions. Once, when he went to the home of one of his grandfather's friends and found him drinking rakı (the distilled alcoholic drink of Turkey), he said: "Selmi, we used to drink rakı together, so give me a little now." On another occasion Muhittin met a man familiarly known as Uncle Halis and said to him: "Do you see, Uncle Halis, that before, I was big and you were small. Now it is the opposite. You are big and I am small."

Although Muhittin showed a strong desire for alcohol as a young child, he had not, during his short life, become an excessive drinker of alcohol. At the age of 20 he killed himself when depressed over a marriage into which he believed he was being forced.

Susumu Ogura was born in Niigata, Japan, on March 21, 1944. At his birth he was found to have a crescent-shaped birthmark behind his right ear. On the basis of this birthmark and it alone, he was identified as the reincarnation of his older brother Shizuo, who had died, probably of pneumonia, after an operation for the drainage of the cells behind and above the right ear. This operation, called mastoidectomy, was often performed in the 1930s (before the development of antibiotics) on patients with severe infections of the middle ear and adjoining cells, called the mastoid cells. The surgeon made a crescent-shaped incision for this operation. Shizuo died on April 20, 1939, at the age of about 18 months.

I have not yet been able to meet Susumu Ogura, and the photographs of his birthmark that I have were sent to me by his brother, Dr. Tadao Ogura, and Tosio Kasahara. In adulthood, Susumu's birthmark remained crescent-shaped, although it had shown some migration (away from the ear) as he grew up. It was a hairless, slightly elevated area behind the right ear and measured about 3 centimeters long and 5 millimeters wide at its widest (Figure 8).

Susumu never made any statements about the life of his older brother, who had died in infancy.

Because Susumu's mother was well aware of the operation on Shizuo, this case might be interpreted as an instance of a maternal impression. A difficulty with this interpretation, however, arises from the birth of a male baby, Takashi, who was born between the death of Shizuo and Susumu's birth. One might have expected that a maternal impression, if it played a role, would have produced a birthmark on Takashi, but he had none.

Jacinta Agbo, an Igbo of Nigeria, was born in 1980. She had the most extra-ordinary birthmark that I have ever seen. It consisted of an area, about 3 centimeters wide, of pale, scarlike tissue that extended around her entire head (Figure 9). In some respects it resembled a bandage, and I believe it did in fact correspond in location to a bandage placed around the head of the deceased person with whom Jacinta was later identified.

This person, Nsude Agbo, had been engaged in a quarrel during which one of the combatants hit him on the head with a club. He was taken to the University

Hospital in Enugu and operated upon. I was unable to obtain copies of the medical record of this operation which occurred in March 1970. (Many of the medical records in the University Hospsital had been mislaid or destroyed during the Biafran War, which lasted from 1967 to 1970.) It is safe to assume, however, that a neurosurgeon attempted to prize up the battered-in skull bones of Nsude. In order to do this he would first have made an extensive incision in the scalp, which he would afterward have sewn up. Jacinta's birthmark was much wider than the incision would have been, and this is why I believe it corresponded to a bandage placed by the surgeon around the head after he had sewn up the scalp.

This is a case of the sex-change type. When I met Jacinta, she was only 2 years old. One of my assistants in Nigeria was able to make follow-up visits to her, first when she was 4 and again when she was almost 8 years old. He learned that she had shown definitely masculine traits. She thought of herself as a boy and "did everything that they [boys] do." Her birthmark had not faded; if anything, it had become more prominent.

Maung Nyunt Win was a member of a small crowd observing my assistant and me as we were studying another case in his village in Upper Burma. I noticed the enormous hairy nevus on his cheek (Figure 10) and thought this might derive from a previous life. We called him over and learned that this was indeed so. Later, we were able to interview several informants for the case.

The informants told us that Maung Nyunt Win's hairy nevus corresponded to what I believe was a sebaceous cyst at the same location on the cheek of the man, U Po Hla, whose life Maung Nyunt Win remembered. Such cysts tend to enlarge and become unsightly and sometimes uncomfortable. U Po Hla decided to drain the cyst himself. After puncturing it with a pin or needle, he squeezed out its contents. Miraculously, he did not infect the cyst, and he lived some years longer before he died of some unrelated illness. He had not, however, fully abolished all trace of the cyst; some kind of scar must have remained after the drainage.

Maung Nyunt Win made a few statements showing that he had some imaged memories of the life of U Po Hla.

James Wilder, a member of the Gitksan tribe of British Columbia, was born in Kitwancool, British Columbia, Canada, on June 13, 1938. At his birth he was found to have a large, heavily pigmented nevus in his left upper abdomen. In adulthood, when I met him, it measured approximately 3 centimeters by 1.5 centimeters (*).

James's mother, Gertrude, perhaps had an announcing dream before his birth. He himself had only some vague possible memories that might or might not have derived from a previous life. He was, nevertheless, identified as the reincarnation of James McIntosh, who had died of an abdominal cancer, probably of the stomach, on August 27, 1931. The cancer had been neglected or was considered inoperable when James first consulted a doctor. Before he died, it eroded the abdominal wall, where a fistula developed. James Wilder's birthmark was at the location of this fistula.

Ma Khin Sandi was born in Rangoon, Burma, on September 9, 1983. Her parents were U Hla Shein and Ma Omar. Before Ma Khin Sandi's birth her mother had a strong impression that her mother, Daw Khin Mya, was to be reborn as her baby and would have birthmarks on her back and left wrist.

Daw Khin Mya had died on November 16, 1979, at the age of 50. She had suffered from hypertension for many years. Some months before her death she had had a stroke with paralysis of her right side and became bedridden. From lying more or less helpless on her back she developed a bedsore in the lower back.

When Ma Khin Sandi was born, she was found to have a birthmark on her lower back at the site of the bedsore from which Daw Khin Mya had suffered (*). It was a small, triangular area of increased pigmentation and measured (when Ma Khin Sandi was an infant) about 1 centimeter by 5 millimeters.

Ma Khin Sandi had another birthmark. This was a small round area of increased pigmentation on the upper surface of her left wrist (*). It corresponded to a mark that someone had made at this site on the body of Daw Khin Mya, either as she was dying or soon after her death. This birthmark was of the type that I call "experimental birthmarks," and I will delay a further discussion of them until Chapter 10, where I shall describe other examples.

I met Ma Khin Sandi first when she was an infant in arms and then again when she was about 2½ years old. She was then just beginning to use pencils and crayons. Watching her draw, I noticed that she was using her left hand. All the other members of the family were right-handed. Daw Khin Mya had also been right-handed. She, however, had lost the use of her right hand after her stroke. I have asked myself whether Ma Khin Sandi's left-handedness might derive from a residue of Daw Khin Mya's inability during the last months of her life to use her right hand. In Chapter 23 I describe some other cases in which left-handedness seemed to derive from a previous life.

Bir Sahai belonged to a group of older subjects in India whose cases Dr. Satwant Pasricha and I investigated together in the 1970s. We wanted to learn whether Indian cases two generations apart would have similar features, and we found that they had. Bir Sahai, like many of the other subjects of this group, lived in a relatively inaccessible village. It was not the village of his birth. That was a place called Saunhar in the Etah District of Uttar Pradesh, India. He was born into the Chamar caste, one of the lowest in India. As often occurs with subjects of Bir Sahai's generation (and social class), no written records fixed the date of his birth, and he himself could not state it accurately. From various indications we settled on 1912 as a plausible year for his birth. When Bir Sahai was born, he had a large, scarlike birthmark on his back, and I shall describe that later.

It happened that a circuit judge had learned of Bir Sahai's case in the 1920s (when Bir Sahai was a youth). The judge had made some inquiries about the case from firsthand witnesses and wrote a report of it that eventually came to me. To supplement this information, Dr. Pasricha and I found some older persons still living and still able to remember something of how the case developed; this group included Bir Sahai himself.

I did not learn how old Bir Sahai had been when it first occurred to him that somehow he was a Thakur (a much higher caste than that of the Chamars) and did not belong in the village where he had been born; but his first communication of this information occurred when he was about 4, when a Thakur in the village ordered Bir Sahai's mother to perform some menial task, such as, perhaps, to collect cow dung for fuel. Bir Sahai protested at this; from his childish perspective he was a Thakur himself and therefore his mother must also be one and should be treated respectfully. This was not the view of the Thakur who had ordered Bir Sahai's mother to do some work, and he roundly abused Bir Sahai. Thereupon, Bir Sahai said that he would send for some of his people from Nardauli, who would punish the Thakur for his impertinence. The other villagers then asked Bir Sahai to explain his connection with Nardauli, which he did.

Bir Sahai said that he was a native of Nardauli (another village of the Etah District, northwest of Etah, about 40 kilometers from Saunhar). He said that he was Thakur Megh Singh. Megh Singh's mother was still living then, and when she learned of Bir Sahai's statements, she sent for him to come to Nardauli. There, he recognized her and also recognized Megh Singh's gun and spear as well as two other persons known to Megh Singh. Bir Sahai's statements impressed Megh Singh's family so much that they thereupon adopted him. He moved to Nardauli and spent the rest of his life there; it was there that we met him.

Caste is still a serious matter in India, but it was even more so during the first decades of this century, when Bir Sahai was a child and youth. When Megh Singh's family adopted Bir Sahai, they probably assumed that the other Thakurs of Nardauli would accept him like one of themselves, as they did. It did not work out that way. The other Thakurs of Nardauli regarded Bir Sahai as a Chamar (which he was by birth), and they would not marry their daughters to him. He, for his part, regarded himself as a Thakur (from the previous life), and he would not marry a girl of a lower caste. Thus he remained a bachelor all his life, a social prisoner, we might say, of the caste system in India. Even so, he was certainly better off economically among a family of prosperous landowners in Nardauli than he would have been if he had remained among the impoverished Chamars of Saunhar.

I come now to Bir Sahai's birthmark. The judge who wrote the first report of the case in the 1920s excited my interest in finding Bir Sahai by mentioning that he had personally seen "a big scar near the spine of Bir Sahai. This is the scar of the carbuncle from which Megh Singh had died." Nearly 50 years later Dr. Pasricha and I were able to examine and photograph this "scar." Its description with the word *scar* did not seem inappropriate, because it closely resembled the sort of scar that a furuncle or carbuncle might leave if it healed. It was ovoid in shape, but somewhat irregularly so. It was approximately 3 centimeters long and 2 centimeters wide. It was a reddish purple. The center was slightly depressed and darker than the peripheral area (*).

According to Bir Sahai, the birthmark had not discharged when he was born. Nor had its appearance changed since then. (He could not have seen it himself, but he would have been informed by older persons, if this had happened.) He had never had any pain or other discomfort in the area of the birthmark.

It remains to consider why Bir Sahai, a Chamar of Saunhar, should have had the memories of a Thakur of Nardauli. If we are willing to consider reincarnation as a plausible interpretation of the case, an answer presents itself. An informant in Saunhar told us that Megh Singh's wife came from Malawan, which is the nearest town of any substance to Saunhar. Bir Sahai's memories of the previous life had included the detail that Megh Singh's wedding party (when it was coming to Malawan) had camped under some trees outside the village of Saunhar. If we add to this information the detail that Megh Singh's widow might have moved back to her village after his death—as many widows do in India—and suppose that a discarnate Megh Singh wanted to remain near her, we can imagine that the discarnate Megh Singh got himself "accidentally reborn," so to speak, to Bir Sahai's mother. This line of reasoning provides another example of what I call the "geographical factor" as a hypothesis to understand cases like Bir Sahai's in which, at first examination, there seems no reason for a child in one village to have memories about a life in another and remote one. I gave another example of the geographical factor in my report of the case of Maung Aye Kyaw in Chapter 4. Interested readers can find additional examples in some of my other books.

8

BIRTHMARKS CORRESPONDING TO OTHER TYPES OF WOUNDS OR MARKS ON DECEASED PERSONS

In this chapter I describe a heterogeneous group of cases that illustrate further the variety of wounds and other marks to which birthmarks may correspond. The deaths of the previous personalities in these cases were all natural, and the relevant wounds or marks had no connection with the deaths, as they had in all but one of the cases of the preceding four chapters.

Santosh Sukla was born in the village of Panchwati, Uttar Pradesh, India, on July 3, 1950. A girl called Maya had said before her death that she was going to be reborn to Santosh's parents. The two families were acquainted and distantly related. When Santosh became able to speak, she spoke abundantly about the life of Maya. Her statements and some recognitions of persons and places familiar to Maya convinced the members of both families that she was the reincarnation of Maya.

Santosh had markedly visible red lines in the outer surfaces (sclerae) of her eyes; they were in fact abnormally dilated small arteries (arterioles). Maya had

had similarly prominent red lines in her eyes. She and Santosh were the only members of the families with this abnormality. The dilated arterioles were still sufficiently prominent when Santosh was 25 years old in 1975, so that I was able to photograph them (*).

Savitri Devi Pathak was born on June 5, 1947, in the village of Ahmedpur, which is in the Mainpuri District of Uttar Pradesh, India. Her family were Brahmins. When Savitri Devi was born, her mother noted that one of her finger-nails was black; but she attached no importance to this abnormality until Savitri Devi began to speak about a previous life. Savitri Devi did not do this until the comparatively late age of 5 years. (She had begun to speak much earlier, at between 2 and 2½ years of age.)

Savitri Devi said that she had a house in Shikohabad (a small city about 15 kilometers east of Ahmedpur) and belonged to a family of Dhobis (the caste of washermen). She gave no name for the person whose life she seemed to remem-ber, nor for that of her (previous) father. She referred, however, to one "Minminia" (without explaining who this person was) and to a brother called Nadaria. She explained the mark on her nail by saying that in the previous life a weight (from a balance used for weighing grain) had dropped on her thumb and left a permanent bruise. When someone asked Savitri Devi how she had died, she replied that she had died after drinking some red water drawn from a well.

Despite the paucity of proper names that Savitri Devi had stated, her uncle Komal Singh thought that he could solve the case by making inquiries among the washermen at Shikohabad. (The task was made easier by the tendency of urban mem-bers of the same caste in India to inhabit the same quarter of a town or city.) He found a family of washermen having a member, Puniya, whose nickname was "Minminia." (The name means "one who speaks through her nose"; Puniya had a cleft palate.) This family had lost a daughter, Munni, some years earlier, and Munni had had her left thumbnail injured some time before her death when a weight had accidentally fallen on it. She had been left with a permanent blackness of the nail, called in medicine a subungual hematoma. Munni's black fingernail was well remembered in her family. One informant told us that Munni's parents had said, when they heard about Savitri Devi: "If she has a mark on her left thumb, then she is our child."

The blackness of Savitri Devi's left thumbnail persisted at least until 1974, when she was 27 years old. I photographed it in that year (*).

Ma Chit Chit Than was born in Mandalay, Burma, on June 21, 1971. Before her birth her mother, Daw Than, had a dream that prepared her to expect the rebirth of one of her daughters, Ma Khin San Tin, who had died about a year earli-er, at the age of about 4.

When Ma Chit Chit Than was born, her parents noted that she had a red birthmark on the upper eyelid of her right eye and the surrounding area of her forehead above the right eye. This birthmark corresponded in location to some medicine that Daw Than had accidentally spilled on the face of Ma Khin San Tin when the girl was on the point of dying. Daw Than had been trying to put some red medicine into her dying daughter's mouth, but she was so distraught by the child's condition that she spilled the medicine on the child's eye and forehead. Daw Than then tried to wipe the medicine off her daughter's face, but much of it remained when, a few minutes later, Ma Khin San Tin died. Daw Than thought that the red medicine might generate a birthmark on a later-born daughter who could thus be recognized. Ma Khin San Tin was therefore buried with the residue of the red medicine still on her face.

When Ma Chit Chit Than became able to speak, she had some memories of the life of Ma Khin San Tin. These included the moments before death, when Daw Than had spilled medicine on her face.

Ma Chit Chit Than's birthmark was a port-wine stain that, as I mentioned, covered an extensive area of her right upper eyelid and adjacent parts of her forehead (Figure 11). I photographed it first when she was not quite 6 years old and again 7 years later, when she was 12½ years old (*). Like most port-wine stains, hers had not faded as she grew older.

John Rose, a Tlingit, was born in Angoon, Alaska, on October 5, 1963. At birth he had a somewhat faint birthmark on the back of his left hand. On the basis of this birthmark and an announcing dream, he was identified as the reincarnation of William Paul (a great-uncle of his mother), who had had the head of a wolf tattooed on the back of his hand. The birthmark on John Rose did not show much of the wolf's head, but I could easily discern a part that corresponded to one of the wolf's ears, and I sketched that (*).

Linda Chijioke, an Igbo, was born on September 16, 1981, in a village near Ndeaboh, Anambra State, Nigeria. Almost immediately after Linda's birth, her parents noticed that she had a large birthmark of blue-black pigmentation at the top of her head. It covered about one quarter of the surface area of the upper part of the scalp (*). Her parents thought this might be from some disease and consulted a doctor without obtaining any help from him. They had given Linda the name of a deceased person—on what basis I did not learn—but Linda became ill, and they thought they might have made a mistake in naming her. (The Igbo often attribute illnesses in infants to misnaming.) They consulted an oracle, who told them that Linda was in fact the reincarnation of her paternal grandmother, Ori Chijioke, who had died in 1967. He explained Linda's birthmark as a residue from abrasions on the skin resulting from carrying heavy loads on the head.

All Nigerian women of the villages carry loads on their heads. There were two aspects of Ori's carrying such loads, however, in which she differed from most other Nigerian village women. First, her husband was a trader over long distances, and his wife accompanied him on his trading journeys, which were made on foot. She carried on her head some of the goods to be traded, and, on the way back, she carried the money her husband had earned. In the days of his trading the currency was an ingot of heavy metal called an *okpoo*, and a successful trading journey meant that on the way home Ori carried on her head a heavy load of these ingots. The second distinctive feature in Ori's circumstances was her attitude toward carrying such heavy loads on her head. She was happily married, and she never openly grumbled about having to carry heavy loads on her head. One informant, however, remembered that Ori had told her privately that she did not intend to suffer in this way—meaning from carrying heavy loads on her head—in her next incarnation.

Some Nigerian women develop abrasions and even blisters at the tops of their heads, where the loads they carry sit; and Ori had had such a lesion at the top of her head. Birthmarks related to such lesions, however, occur rarely. (I learned of some others, but Linda's was the only one I saw.) The Igbo interpretation of Linda's birthmark attributed it to Ori's "rejection of one's lot in life." This means that her discontent with carrying loads on her head, although mostly tacit, had generated Linda's birthmark.

When Linda became able to speak, she showed a strong identification with Ori and asked to be called Ori. She made only a few statements about the life of Ori. When asked about the birthmark on the top of her head, she said that it came from the life of Ori. Unlike other Nigerian children of her age, she did not play at carrying loads on her head. When the other children in playing would put something on their heads and carry it in this way, she would carry her load in her hands.

I have investigated the cases of nine subjects who had birthmarks on their ears that informants said corresponded to holes in the previous personalities' ears which had been pierced for earrings. Of these subjects, two were in India, three in Burma, one in Sri Lanka, and three in British Columbia, Canada. The informants sometimes said that when a subject had been born, there had been a hole entirely through the helix of the ear; but these had later closed up. Some of the birthmarks I examined still had small pits as well as increased pigmentation; others had only increased pigmentation. I examined and photographed all of these myself (*), except for 1 subject in Burma whose birthmark I sketched (*) and 2 subjects in British Columbia whom I was unable to meet; from informants' descriptions I made sketches of the birthmarks on these last 2 subjects (*). To complete this chapter, I will summarize the case of the subject in British Columbia whose birthmarks I examined and photographed.

Edward Taylor, a member of the Gitksan tribe, was born in Hazelton, British Columbia, Canada, on November 26, 1973. Edward was born with birthmarks at the back of the helix of each ear. The marks were areas of increased pigmentation;

and they were slightly depressed below the level of the surrounding skin (Figures 12 and 13).

A resident of Hazelton, Patrick Carter, had died the year before Edward's birth after predicting that he would reincarnate and stay in the home of a relative, Jean Slade, of whom he was fond; Edward was this man's great-nephew. At the age of 4 Edward moved to Jean Slade's house and seems to have spent much of his childhood there.

Patrick Carter's ears had been pierced for earrings when he was young, and Edward's birthmarks were considered evidence that Patrick had reincarnated as planned. When Edward became able to speak, he made a few statements and showed behavior suggestive of his having memories of Patrick Carter's life.

9

NEVI CORRESPONDING TO WOUNDS OR OTHER MARKS ON DECEASED PERSONS

Although nearly all the birthmarks that I have so far described were not ordinary moles or nevi, a few definitely were of this type. For example, the birthmark on U Tinn Sein (described in Chapter 4) was a flat round area of increased pigmentation and thus what a dermatologist would call a hyperpigmented macule, a type of nevus. We could say the same of some other birthmarks I have described in earlier chapters, such as that of Susan Wilson.

In this chapter of the monograph I consider the cases of 14 other subjects each of whom had a birthmark that we could describe as a nevus. This uses the word *nevus* somewhat loosely, because the birthmarks included in this chapter were often much larger than the ordinary nevi familiar to dermatologists. In eight of these cases, the subject's birthmark corresponded to a wound or other mark on the previous personality's body. In the other six cases, the birthmark corresponded to a similar nevus on the previous personality.

Among the six cases in which a nevus on the subject corresponded to one on the previous personality, the subject and previous personality were related in all but one case. When this circumstance occurs, we need to consider the possibility that a genetic factor may account for the recurrence of the nevus in the same location in a second member of the family. We can say that, in general, genetic factors play a minor role in the number of nevi that a person has. (Exceptions occur in certain diseases, such as von Recklinghausen's Disease.) Genetic factors seem even less important in determining the location of nevi at particular sites of the body. Even so, a few pedigrees have been published in which the facts suggested inheritance for the site of a nevus. Moreover, in families thus affected, occasionally one generation may be skipped with the reappearance of a nevus at the same site in a later generation.

The acknowledgment of a genetic factor in the occurrence of a nevus at a particular location does not exclude the influence of other factors, including some from a previous life. It is legitimate to ask why, if a nevus is inherited at a particular location, one particular member of the family has it, but other members do not. To illustrate this point I will present brief accounts of two cases of this group.

Cemal Kurt was born in Yenice, Turkey, in 1961. Before his birth a neighbor had a dream which was interpreted as meaning that a distant relative of the Kurts, Cemal Karacan, would be reborn in their family. Without questioning this, Cemal's parents named him after this relative. Cemal Kurt had a prominent port-wine stain birthmark on his left forearm (Figure 14), but his parents only learned later that Cemal Karacan had had a similar birthmark. They also only learned later that one of Cemal Karacan's sons had also had a dream indicating that his father would be reborn in the Kurt family. When Cemal was about 2 years old, he began to speak and soon started referring to a previous life. He said that he owned a vineyard, and he made a few other statements and recognitions appropriate for Cemal Karacan. The sons of Cemal Karacan accepted him as their father reborn and got into the habit of calling him "Father" before he was even 5 years old. One of these sons was a barber, and for many years he cut Cemal's hair without charging him. Cemal for his part showed unusual fondness for Cemal Karacan's wife, Elif; and he was much affected when she died, even though by that time he had forgotten the imaged memories he had earlier had of the previous life.

Maung Sein Nyunt was born in Bassein, Lower Burma, on November 18, 1957. His parents were U Hla Maung and his wife, Daw Mya Mya.

U Hla Maung had a younger brother, U Khin Tin. He was a robust young man of about 30 when he drowned accidentally in one of the lakes in Rangoon. He somewhat impulsively went for a swim alone, crossed the lake, and then developed cramps as he was swimming back. He drowned before help could reach him.

About 15 months later, in July 1957, Daw Mya Mya dreamed on three successive nights that her deceased brother-in-law, U Khin Tin, came and stood at the foot of her bed. The dreams were vivid and somewhat frightening. Daw Mya Mya told her husband about the dreams, and he interpreted them as indicating that his brother would be reborn as their son. At the time, this was not a welcome prospect to Daw Mya Mya.

As soon as Maung Sein Nyunt was born, U Hla Maung examined him and found that he had on his left back a large area of increased pigmentation (*), which closely resembled in size and location a similar area that U Khin Tin had had.

Maung Sein Nyunt never spoke about the life of his uncle, although in his family of Burmese Buddhists he would certainly have been allowed to do so, if he had wished. He did, however, have a severe phobia of water. It persisted until he was about 15 or 16 years old. When I met him and photographed his birthmark, he was 19½ years old. He said that he was then able to swim, but did not much enjoy doing so.

As an infant Maung Sein Nyunt cried whenever his mother held him, but he was content in his father's arms. This unusual behavior eventually reminded Daw Mya Mya that after she had dreamed of her brother-in-law she had initially wished that he would not be reborn in their family. It occurred to her that if Maung Sein Nyunt was the reincarnation of U Khin Tin, he might be annoyed at her attitude toward him. She therefore held the baby in her arms and, speaking aloud, apologized to him and said that he was welcome in their family. After that, Maung Sein Nyunt did not cry when his mother held him. He was then about 8 months old.

The size of this work prevents me from describing other cases of nevi that I include in the monograph. I do not wish to leave the subject, however, without using the variety of nevi that is found among the birthmarks to emphasize what I already mentioned in Chapter 2: Differences in the subjects' skins seem to be important determinants of the kind of birthmark that may correspond to a wound, nevus, or other mark on a deceased person. From the cases already described and to be described, one can see that similar types of birthmarks (for example, ones with increased pigmentation) may correspond to different types of wounds. On the other hand, different types of birthmarks may correspond to similar types of wounds. For example, burns in one case (Ma Khin Hsann Oo) corresponded to multiple elevated, hairy areas of increased pigmentation and in another (Patricia Fairley) to a port-wine stain birthmark. In the case of Hanumant Saxena a birthmark having decreased pigmentation corresponded to a shotgun wound; but in the cases of Obike Nwonye and Ma Mu Mu birthmarks corresponding to shotgun wounds were depressed scarlike areas with no change in pigmentation of the skin.

In the monograph I give two long tables with additional examples that illustrate even more fully the point I wish to make here: We cannot predict what kind of birthmark may derive from a particular type of injury, and from examining a birthmark we can only rarely say to what kind of injury it corresponds. I consider some exceptions to this last statement in Chapter 12, which I devote to a discussion, with examples, of the unusual details observed in some of the birthmarks.

10

THE PREDICTION OF
BIRTHMARKS

The simplest type of prediction of birthmarks states that an already existing birthmark will be found if looked for in a certain place on a subject's body. The birthmark exists, but has not been noticed, mentioned, or verified. In Chapter 8 I gave a simple example of this kind of prediction in citing the remark of Munni's parents about Savitri Devi: "If she has a mark on her left thumb, she is our child." I will describe three predictions of this type in this chapter.

A second type of prediction occurs when a person (usually an elderly one) selects parents for his or her next incarnation and specifies details, such as a birthmark, by which surviving relatives may recognize him or her in the new incarnation. I will describe one example of this type of prediction in this chapter and include another example in Chapter 12.

A third type of prediction involves the marking of a dying or recently dead person with some substance, such as charcoal. The mark is put at a particular location, and later-born children (of the extended family or area) are examined to see whether they have a birthmark at the site of the marking. As I mentioned in Chapter 7, I call these cases instances of experimental birthmarks. That is perhaps a slightly extravagant term, but yet not altogether inappropriate, because the person marking the body hopes to control the location of a birthmark on a baby not yet born. I have some information on 20 examples of experimental birthmarks, but space in this chapter will permit brief accounts of only a few of these. Before coming to these, I shall present summaries of three cases of the first type of prediction and one case of the second type.

Cemil Fahrici was born in Antakya, Hatay, Turkey, in 1935. During the night before Cemil's birth, his father, Mikail Fahrici, dreamed that a distant relative, Cemil Hayik, entered his house. Cemil Hayik had just recently been killed under circumstances that I shall describe, and his appearance in the dream prepared Cemil's parents to believe that Cemil Hayik would be reborn as their son. This belief became stronger when they noticed a prominent birthmark under Cemil's right chin (Figure 15). It was a scarlike area that bled for some days after his birth; his parents took him to a hospital, where the wound was stitched.

Cemil Hayik had been a picturesque bandit whose troubles began when he killed two men who had raped two of his sisters. Although arrested for these murders, he contrived to escape, and for about 2 years he maintained a precarious freedom in the sparsely inhabited mountainous area between the cities of Antakya and Samandağ. It was not difficult for him to stop travelers in that isolated region and rob them of whatever he needed. In those days (the early 1930s) France occupied the province of Hatay, which Turkey was trying to recover; and the mountain people probably gave only limited assistance to the French police hunting Cemil Hayik. Eventually, he and his brother (who had joined him) were betrayed, and the French police surrounded the house in which the brothers had taken refuge. A conventional shoot-out occurred, until finally the police were able to approach closely enough to pour gasoline on the house and set it on fire. As the fire consumed the house, the shots from inside ceased. Then the silence was broken by two more shots, and a further silence ensued. Cautiously, the police approached the house and kicked the door open. Inside, they found the bodies of Cemil Hayik and his brother. It appeared that Cemil Hayik had first killed his brother and then, putting the muzzle of his gun to his chin, he had set off the trigger with his toe and killed himself. The bullet entered his head beneath the right side of his chin. The bodies of the bandit brothers were taken into Antakya and displayed in the courthouse square, perhaps as a demonstration of French police competence, perhaps as a deterrent to other persons feeling inclined to take up banditry. Cemil Fahrici was born a few days after Cemil Hayik died.

When Cemil Fahrici became able to speak—from the age of about 2 on—he described "bit by bit" the life and death of Cemil Hayik. Cemil had imaged memories of the previous life when awake; and he also had nightmarish dreams about fighting the French police. These persisted until he was between 6 and 7 years old. Although his parents—from the dream and Cemil's birthmark—believed that Cemil was probably the reincarnation of Cemil Hayik, they had not initially called him Cemil, but gave him the name "Dahham." Cemil resolutely refused to be called by any name other than Cemil, and his parents eventually yielded to his demand.

As a child Cemil had a markedly hostile attitude toward policemen and would throw stones at them and also at soldiers. He would play with a stick as if it were a rifle; and he once tried to take his father's rifle and shoot some soldiers with it. Despite his militant postures toward the police, Cemil suffered from a phobia of blood. He developed friendly relations with Cemil Hayik's family and exchanged gifts with them.

For several years while investigating this case I believed that Cemil Fahrici had only one birthmark. Then one of Cemil Hayik's sisters, during an interview, mentioned that the bullet which had killed her brother had exited at the top of his skull and lifted out a part of its bone. One of the French gendarmes who had been present at the shoot-out ending in Cemil Hayik's death gave a similar description of the exit wound, gesturing with his hands above his head to show how part of Cemil Hayik's skull had been lifted upward by the force of the exiting bullet. When I heard these accounts, I returned to Cemil Fahrici and asked him whether he had another birthmark. Without hesitating he pointed to the top of his head, and we quickly discovered a linear area of hairlessness on the left side of the top of his head (Figure 16). An artist's sketch shows the presumed trajectory of the bullet through Cemil Hayik's head (Figure 17).

Semir Taci was born in Antakya, Turkey, (probably) on July 5, 1945. When I first met him, I was shown marks on his right hand that I was told were birthmarks, although there was some question about whether Semir's parents had noticed them when he was born or only when he began to speak about a previous life.

He was between 3 and 4 years old when he began to do so. He said that he had two mothers, one "large" and one "small." He added that his name was Sekip and that he had a wife and children. As to how he had died, he said that he had been bitten by a poisonous snake on his thumb.

What Semir was saying reminded his parents of a man called Sekip Karşanbaş, who had been raised and befriended by Semir's father. Sekip had been something of a loser. He worked in a café, but he earned little money and spent too much of what he did earn on alcohol. His wife rebuked him for bringing home more alcohol than bread. One day he quarreled with his wife and left the house angrily. He went off to a bakery shop, where someone mentioned that a snake had come into a neighboring shop. Probably intoxicated, Sekip went to the shop and rashly picked up the snake, which bit him. The snake was almost certainly an Ottoman viper, known locally as the "mountain snake." After being bitten, Sekip ran home to his wife with his hand bleeding and was then admitted to the Government Hospital, where he died the following day, on June 24, 1945.

We were able to study the record of Sekip's admission to the Government Hospital in Antakya. It stated that he "had been bitten by a snake on the fingers of the right hand and on those of the left hand." As I mentioned, we had been shown birthmarks on Semir's *right* hand (*), but no one had mentioned birthmarks on his *left* hand. We now examined his left hand and found there marks similar to those on his right hand (*). These marks had a distinctive scarlike appearance; they resembled small keloids, a type of indurated scar with a smooth surface that is raised above the surrounding tissues. All the marks had an identical appearance, and I believe that they were all birthmarks.

Semir had a strong identification with Sekip and frequently said that his name was Sekip. He did not, however, ask to be called by that name. He showed a strong interest in Sekip's children and much affection for them. At first he seemed afraid of Sekip's wife, but as he grew older he became more friendly toward her and enjoyed visiting her. He had a marked phobia of snakes, and this persisted at least until the age of 22, his age when I last met him.

Juggi Lal Agarwal was born in the town of Sirsaganj in the Mainpuri District of Uttar Pradesh, India, on August 13, 1955. His father, Bihari Lal, was a grain dealer. His parents seem not to have noticed any birthmark on him when he was born or soon after.

Not long after Juggi Lal began to speak, he started referring to a previous life. He said that he came from Bhongaon, which is a small town about 65 kilometers north of Sirsaganj. He said that he had been called Puttu Lal and that he had a wife and children in Bhongaon. He further stated that he had been a farmer who brought his grain to Sirsaganj, where he had sold it to Juggi Lal's father. He remembered that unlike many, perhaps most, of the grain dealers of the area, Juggi Lal's father was always scrupulously honest in giving the farmers full value for the grain they brought. He said that he became so attached to Bihari Lal that he thought to himself that if he should die, he would like to be reborn in Bihari Lal's family.

Bihari Lal bought grain from many farmers, and Juggi Lal's statements did not stimulate in him memories of any farmer from Bhongaon whose grain he had bought. He made no move to verify what Juggi Lal was saying. As happens so often in these cases, however, word of what the subject was saying eventually spread back to Bhongaon and reached surviving members of the family of a man called Puttu Lal. These included Puttu Lal's father, Girivar Singh, who decided to go to Sirsaganj and meet Juggi Lal. Upon meeting Juggi Lal he immediately examined the boy's head above his ear and found there what was surely a birthmark. I say this because Juggi Lal had never had any injury at that site; on the other hand, the mark accorded well with the history of Puttu Lal's death.

Puttu Lal had been a peasant farmer (of the Lodha caste) who cultivated his own land. He quarreled with neighbors over the boundaries of their properties. The parties engaged in a fight with heavy batons (called lathis in India). During this engagement one of the combatants struck Puttu Lal on the head. The wound seems then to have become infected, and the infection spread along or under the scalp until it came near the right ear. At this point an abscess either burst spontaneously or was possibly lanced by a doctor who put in a few stitches. After this, the infection must have spread inward, and I conjecture that Puttu Lal died from a severe infection of his blood by bacteria (bacteremia). (At this time and place there were no antibiotics available.) We never succeeded in obtaining fully satisfactory written records of Puttu Lal's injury and medical treatment, although we found fragmentary information about his attendance at different hospitals. I have put together my account of his last illness from these fragments as well as from information I received from surviving members of his family. (These did not include Girivar Singh, who had died by the time we investigated the case.) The point is that Puttu Lal had had some kind of an infection with an opening above his right ear, and the memory of this made his father believe that if Juggi Lal were his son reborn, he should have a birthmark at the same site, which I believe he had. The birthmark, at the time I examined it, consisted of a line somewhat resembling the scar of a small incision; and there seemed to be several tiny punctate scars adjoining it, which might have corresponded to surgical stitch marks (*).

In addition to the statements that I have already mentioned, Juggi Lal made a number of others that proved convincing to the members of Puttu Lal's family. The one that I found most impressive was his statement that his (previous) name (Puttu Lal) had been tattooed on the arm of his daughter. This was nearly correct, but the name tattooed was Puttu *Ram*, not Puttu Lal. I am sure that Juggi Lal could not have obtained this information normally.

Unlike most subjects of these cases, Juggi Lal had no desire to go to Bhongaon and there meet members of the previous family. He was friendly enough with them when they came to meet him; but he had no wish to cultivate close relationships with them. He identified himself with the higher caste of Banias (businessmen) and believed that he should leave behind the lower caste (Lodha) of the previous life.

The subject of the next case, William George, Jr., was a Tlingit. He was born on May 5, 1950, in Juneau, Alaska. During his mother's labor, she had a dream in which her father-in-law, William George, Sr., appeared to her. The dream was so vivid that when she emerged from the anesthetic that she had been given for the delivery, she expected to see her father-in-law, even though she knew, at one level, that he had died about 9 months before.

William George, Sr. had predicted his reincarnation. He told his son Reginald: "If there is anything to this rebirth business, I will come back as your son." He also told his daughter-in-law (Reginald's wife) that when he was reborn he would have birthmarks similar to two that he showed her as he spoke. These were prominent moles, each a little more than half a centimeter in diameter, on the upper surface of his left shoulder and on the upper surface of his left forearm. Later, he again told his son about his plan to reincarnate, and this time he gave his son a gold watch that his mother had given to him. He said: "I'll come back. Keep this watch for me. I am going to be your son." Reginald George took the watch and gave it to his wife, who put it in her jewelry box and kept it there. A few weeks later, in August 1949, William George, Sr. accidentally drowned while fishing from his boat; he had apparently fallen overboard.

When William George, Jr. was born, he was found to have two moles or nevi at the same locations as those of his grandfather, although they were smaller in size (*).

William George, Jr. seems to have spoken little about the life of his grandfather; but his family observed in him several traits in which he resembled his grandfather. He adopted attitudes toward members of the family that would have been appropriate for William George, Sr. (as an older member of the family), but were not for a young boy. His most remarkable statement occurred when he was between 4 and 5 years old. One day his mother decided to lay out on a bed the various objects she had been keeping in her jewelry box. William George, Jr. came into the room and, noticing the watch, picked it up and said: "That's my watch." He clung to it tenaciously and only relinquished it after much persuasion. His mother was convinced that he had never seen the watch before, because she had kept it in the jewelry box ever since her husband had given it to her 5 years before.

As I mentioned in Chapter 9, the location of nevi seems sometimes to be inherited, and a generation may even be skipped in a family with such a genetic trait. (Reginald George had no nevi at the location of his father's.) One may say in this case that because William George, Jr. was a grandson of William George, Sr., he might have inherited the location of the two nevi. There were, however, nine other children in the family besides William George, Jr., and one may reasonably ask why the nevi appeared on his body and not on those of any of the other children of the family.

William George, Sr. had injured his right ankle when he was a young man and was afterward somewhat lame. William George, Jr. had a gait similar to that of his grandfather, which consisted of a tendency to throw his right foot out as he walked. Both his parents commented on the similarity between his gait and that of his grandfather.

I come now to the cases that I have called experimental birthmarks and will describe here two of the numerous cases of this type that we have studied. Then I will briefly summarize three others.

The circumstances leading to the discovery of the first of these three cases strengthened my conviction—mentioned earlier—that the cases are even more frequent than the reports we receive of them lead us to believe. We found the case in the following way. The late Professor Kloom Vajropala of Thailand belonged to a small—almost tiny—group of Asian academics who have become trained in science without disowning the traditions of their culture. Educated at Cambridge and London, Kloom Vajropala eventually became Head of the Department of Biology at Chulalongkorn University in Bangkok. Yet he never ceased to be a devout Buddhist, and he was able to combine his interests in science and religion by accompanying me and assisting me in the investigation of cases in Thailand. One day we were studying a case south of Bangkok. I remarked to him that I thought there were many more cases in Thailand than we had so far learned about. I said there might be one in every village and that they could be found if only someone would look for them. Kloom Vajropala disagreed. I suggested that we go into a nearby village and test my belief. He thought this was a wild idea, but he agreed that we should ask for a case in this village. We went to the village, entered its first boutique (a sort of café), ordered something from the owner, and took our

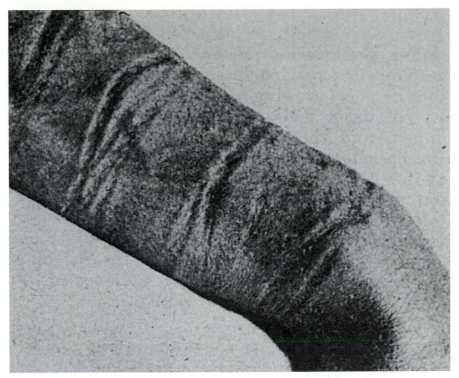

Figure 1 Wheals in the form of rope marks that developed after a patient relived an episode when he had had his arms tied behind his back 9 years earlier. In some of the depressed areas one can notice smaller patterns corresponding to the strands of which the binding rope was made. (Patient of Dr. R. L. Moody.) (Courtesy of *The Lancet*.)

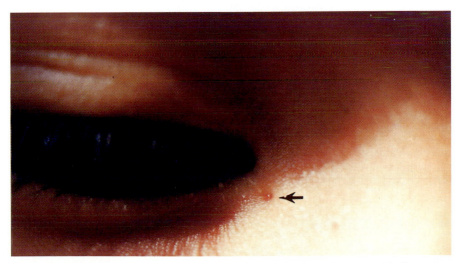

Figure 2 Congenital sinus near the right eye of Calvin Ewing as it appeared in September 1972, when he was 3½ years old.

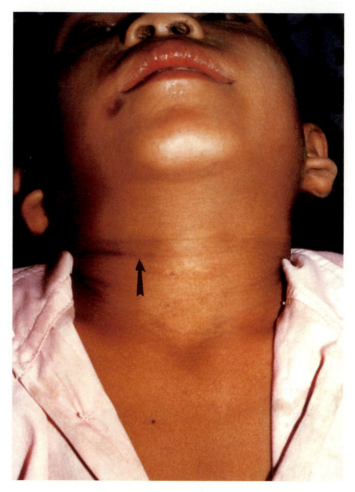

Figure 3 Birthmark on Maung Myint Aung's neck as it appeared in 1980. When the subject's head was tilted back, the birthmark appeared as a linear area of increased pigmentation about 1 centimeter wide extending across the neck.

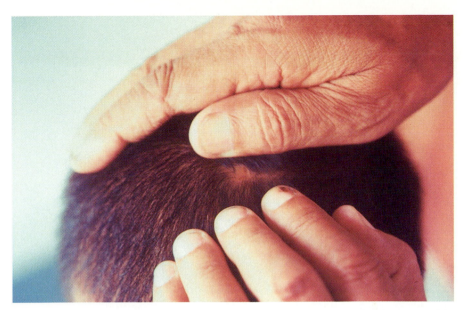

Figure 4 Birthmark at the back of Chanai Choomalaiwong's head as it appeared in March 1979, when he was 11½ years old. It was a round, puckered, hairless area of increased pigmentation, approximately 0.5 centimeter in diameter. This birthmark corresponded to the bullet wound of entry on Bua Kai.

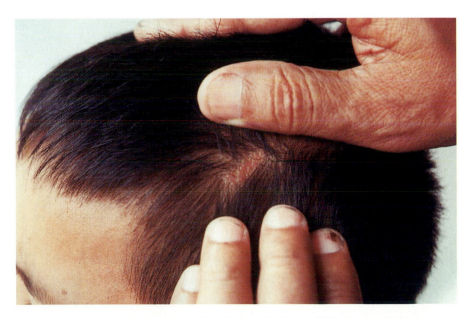

Figure 5 Birthmark at the front of Chanai's head in March 1979. It was a hairless, puckered area of increased pigmentation. It was about 2 centimeters long and 0.5 centimeter wide. This birthmark approximately corresponded (with allowance for some shifting) to the bullet wound of exit on Bua Kai.

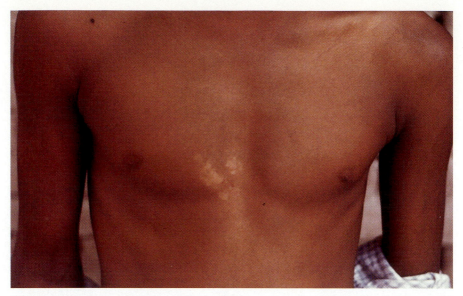

Figure 6 Birthmark on Hanumant Saxena's chest as it appeared in 1971, when he was 16 years old. The birthmark was an area of lessened pigmentation.

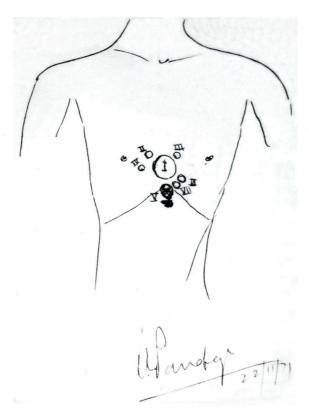

Figure 7 Sketch showing location of fatal wounds on Maha Ram Singh. Dr. S. C. Pandeya (Civil Surgeon, Fatehgarh, U.P., India) drew the circles on the lower chest and upper abdomen. The Roman numerals correspond to the different wounds described in the autopsy report. Number I was the largest wound. Note the characteristic smaller wounds on the periphery of the large, central wound. This is due to the scattering of the shot after they leave the barrel of the gun.

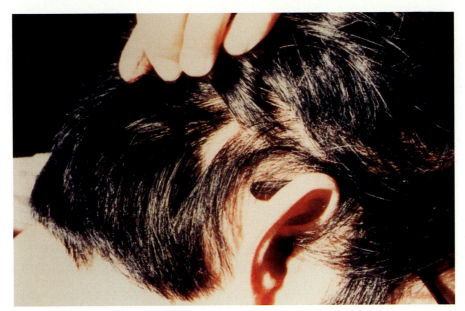

Figure 8 Birthmark on back of the head of Susumu Ogura as it appeared in 1980, when he was 36 years old. The birthmark was a hairless area about 3 centimeters long and 5 millimeters wide. It was shiny and slightly elevated above the surrounding skin. The photograph shows the crescentic shape of the birthmark.

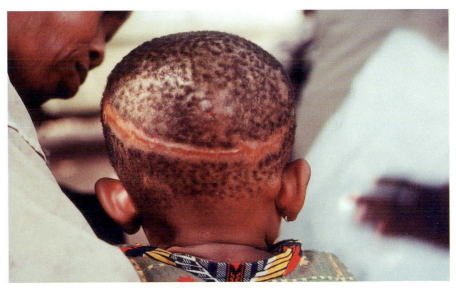

Figure 9 Birthmark on the head of Jacinta Agbo as it appeared in December 1982, when she was just 2 years old. The birthmark was a linear, hairless area extending entirely around the upper part of the head. It had a somewhat uneven, scarlike surface. Its width varied between 2 centimeters and about 3.5 centimeters. This photograph shows the posterior part of Jacinta's head.

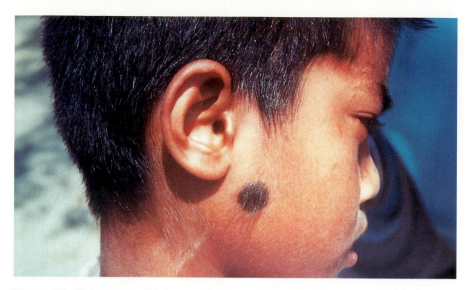

Figure 10 Hairy nevus with increased pigmentation on the right cheek of Maung Nyunt Win when he was approximately 11 years old in 1978. The nevus was round and approximately 1.2 centimeters in diameter.

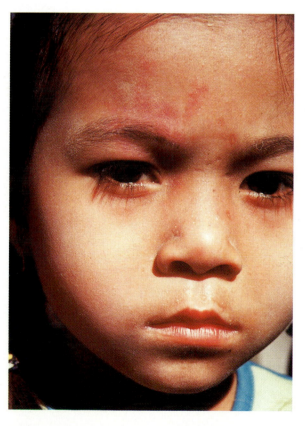

Figure 11 This photograph was taken in March 1977, when Ma Chit Chit Than was about 5½ years old. The birthmark was an area of redness (erythema) covering the right upper eyelid and forehead above the eye.

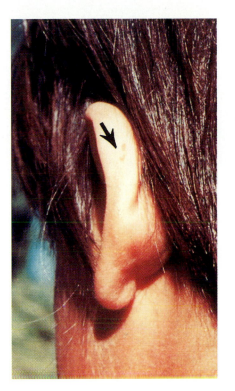 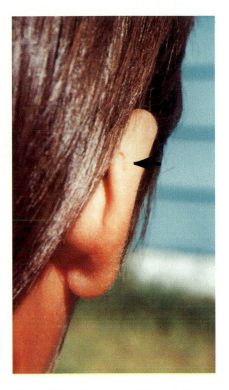

Figure 12 Left ear of Edward Taylor, as it appeared in August 1979, when he was nearly 6 years old. The birthmark was a small depression or pit about 4 millimeters long and 1 millimeter wide. It had increased pigmentation compared with the surrounding skin.

Figure 13 Right ear of Edward Taylor, as it appeared in August 1979, when he was nearly 6 years old. The birthmark resembled that on the left ear, but was less depressed.

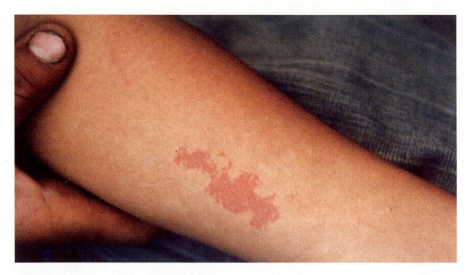

Figure 14 Birthmark, a port-wine stain, on Cemal Kurt's left forearm, as it appeared in September 1975, when he was about 14 years old. The birthmark measured about 4 centimeters by 1.5 centimeters.

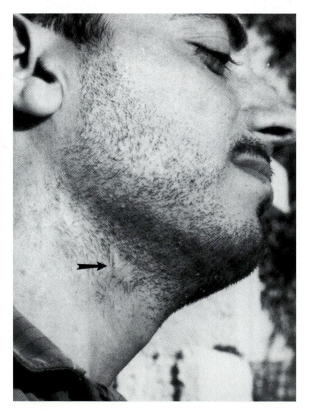

Figure 15 Birthmark on the right upper neck of Cemil Fahrici in 1967, when he was 32 years old. This mark, a hairless scarlike area under the chin, corresponded to the wound of entry on Cemil Hayik. It was about 2 centimeters long and 1 centimeter wide.

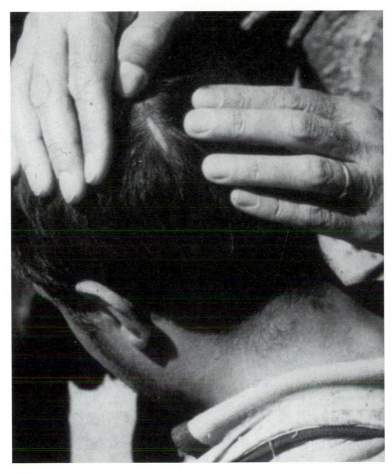

Figure 16 Birthmark on the scalp of Cemil Fahrici in 1970. It was a linear area of hairlessness. This mark corresponded to the wound of exit in Cemil Hayik. It was about 2 centimeters long and 2 millimeters wide.

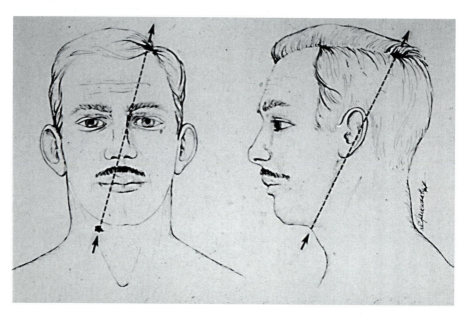

Figure 17 Artist's reconstruction of the trajectory of the bullet through the head of Cemil Hayik that would have caused wounds of entry and exit corresponding to the birthmarks on Cemil Fahrici.

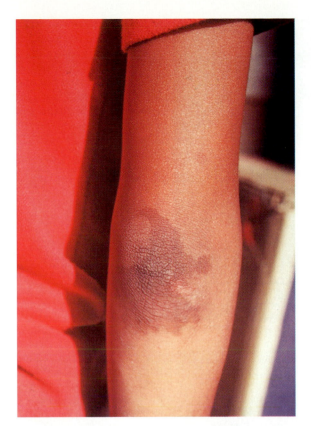

Figure 18 Birthmark on the back of Anurak's elbow as it appeared in March 1978, when he was 8 years old. It was an extensive area of increased pigmentation, irregularly shaped, with dimensions of approximately 5 centimeters wide and 5 centimeters long. The center was almost black.

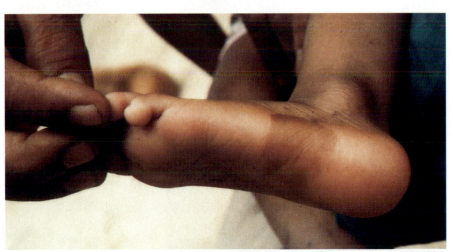

Figure 19 Birthmark on Maung Hla Win's left foot as it appeared when he was 3 years old. The birthmark was an approximately rectangular area of increased pigmentation with dimensions of about 6 centimeters long and 3 centimeters wide. The figure shows how the birthmark extended around the edge of the foot onto the sole.

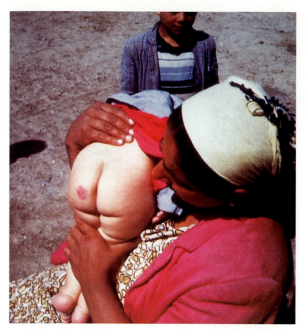

Figure 20 Birthmark on the left buttock of Faris Yuyucuer as it appeared in March 1971, when he was 7 months old. The birthmark was red and slightly puckered. It was generally round in shape and about 1.5 centimeters in diameter.

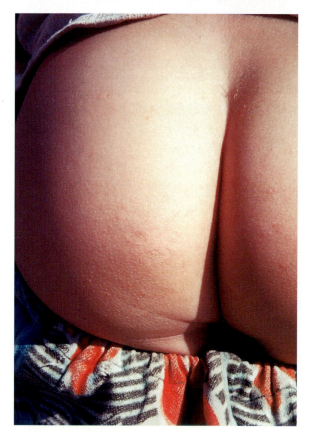

Figure 21 Left buttock of Faris Yuyucuer as it appeared in March 1977, when he was 6½ years old. The birthmark had almost completely disappeared. There was a slight suggestion of increased pigmentation where it had formerly been.

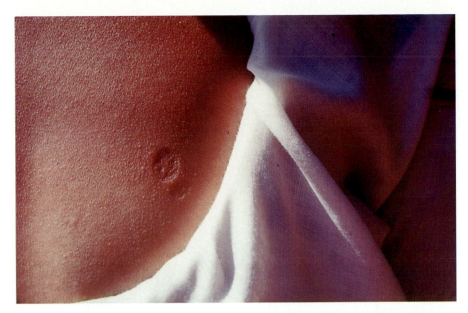

Figure 22 Photograph of the birthmarks on Ma Mu Mu's left breast taken in February 1972, when she was 22½ years old. The birthmarks were both round. The larger one was about 8 millimeters in diameter, the smaller one about 5 millimeters in diameter. Both were depressed below the surrounding skin and puckered.

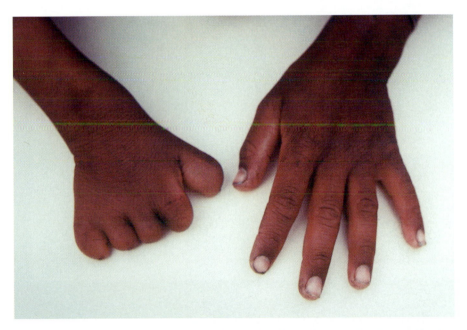

Figure 23 Lekh Pal's hands in February 1980, when he was just over 8 years old. The fingers of the right hand, including the thumb are mere stubs, without any trace of bones. Rudimentary fingernails on three fingers of the right hand cannot be seen in this photograph.

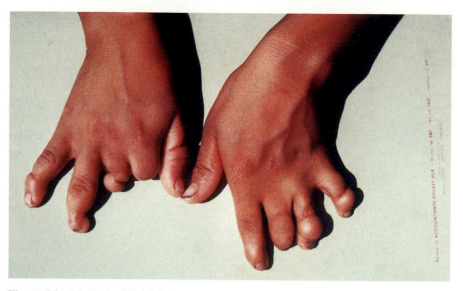

Figure 24   Ma Myint Thein's hands as they appeared in February 1977, when she was 20 years old. All the fingers were markedly shortened and malformed. Most of the fingers and the right thumb showed constriction rings. Only the left thumb was completely normal.

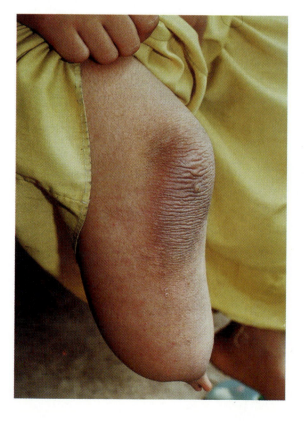

Figure 25   Ma Khin Mar Htoo's right leg as it appeared in 1980, when she was 13 years old. The leg was missing from about 10 centimeters below the knee. Small rudiments of toes protruded from the stump.

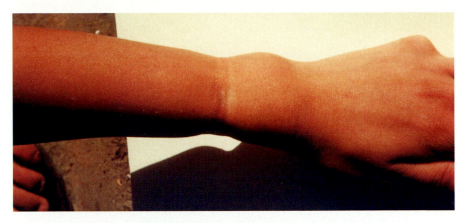

Figure 26 View of Ma Win Tar's left forearm as it appeared in 1978. In this photograph one can see a pattern of three separate depressions extending around the arm and corresponding to the grooves that a rope might make if wrapped tightly around the arm three times.

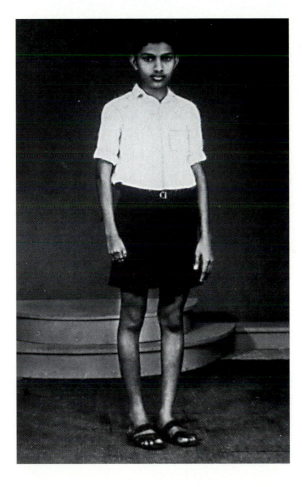

Figure 27 Wijeratne, as he appeared in 1965, when he was 18 years old. His right arm was markedly shorter and underdeveloped compared with his left arm.

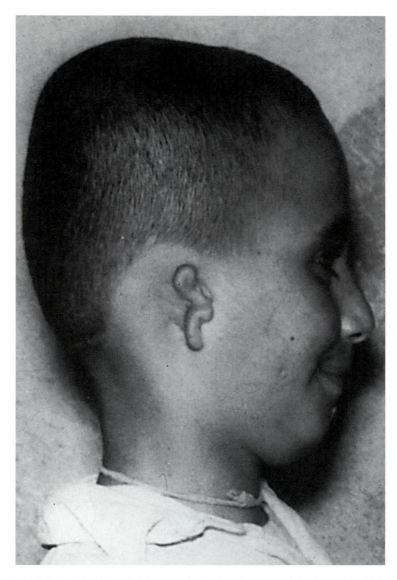

Figure 28 Right side of Semih Tutuşmuş's head as it appeared in November 1967, when he was about 9 years old. The right ear was markedly defective.

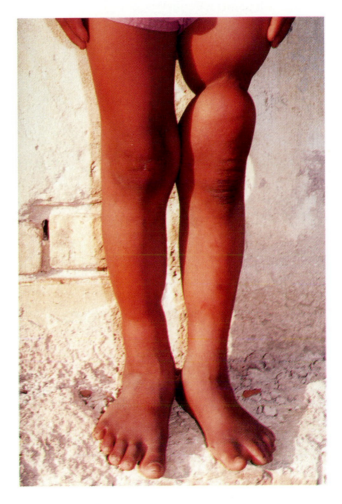

Figure 29 Ma Htwe Win's legs when she was 11 years old. A deep constriction ring can be seen on the left thigh and a more shallow one on the lower part of the right leg. There was a band of increased pigmentation at the same level on the left leg. (The area of this band had formerly been depressed like a constriction ring.)

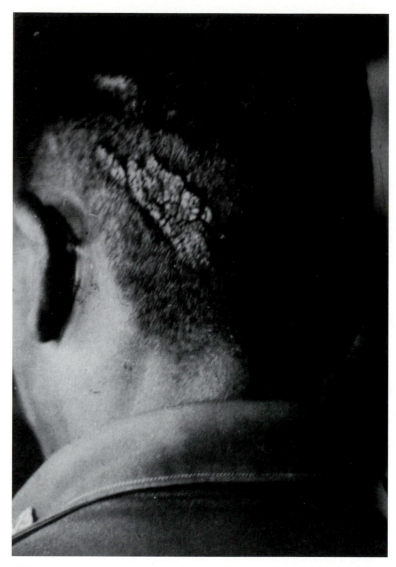

Figure 30 Large nevus, linear and irregular in shape, on the upper part of Thiang San Kla's head. The photograph was taken in January 1963, when he was 38 years old.

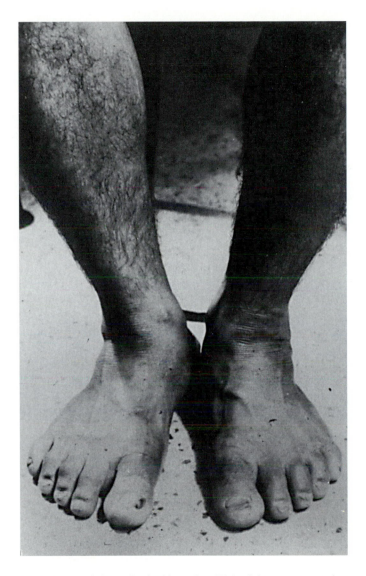

Figure 31 Birth defect of the nail of Thiang San Kla's right great toe as it appeared in March 1969, when he was 44½ years old.

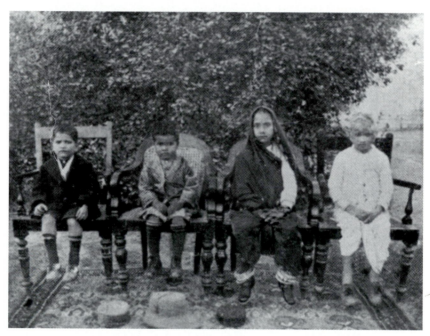

Figure 32 Group of subjects in India who remembered previous lives whose cases K.K.N. Sahay investigated. The photograph was taken in about 1927. B. B. Saxena is the blond boy, wearing a dhoti, seated at the extreme right. At the extreme left is Bishen Chand Kapoor. Next to him (second from the left) is Jagdish Chandra (K.K.N. Sahay's son). The girl is Hira Koer. (Courtesy of Jagdish Chandra.)

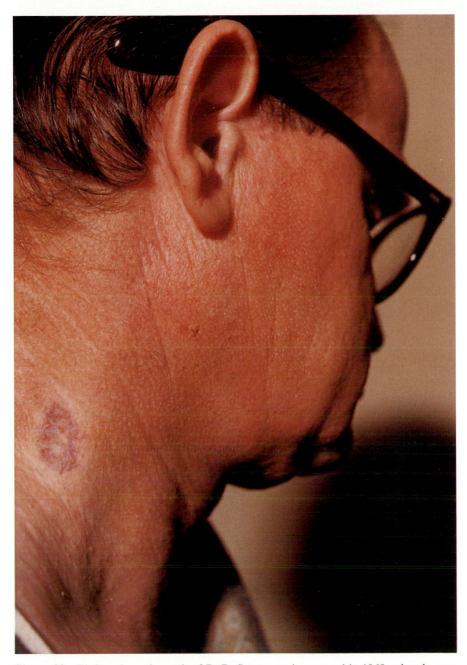

Figure 33 Birthmark on the neck of B. B. Saxena, as it appeared in 1969, when he was about 51 years old. It was roundish and about 2.5 centimeters in diameter. It was an area of erythema, markedly redder than the surrounding skin. The peripheral rim of decreased pigmentation suggests a correspondence of this part of the birthmark to a rim of abraded skin such as frequently occurs around gunshot wounds of entry. (B. B. Saxena's blond hair was dyed brown.)

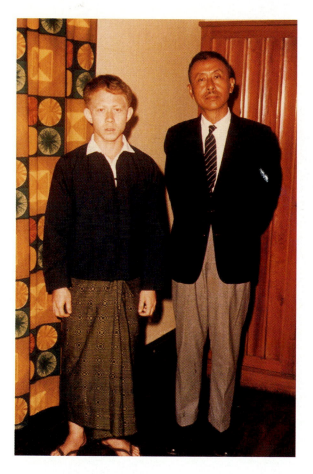

Figure 34 Maung Zaw Win Aung as he appeared in December 1970, when he was about 20½ years old. U Tin Tut (my interpreter) is also shown in the photograph, and readers may compare the pigmentations and forms of the eyes of the two men. Maung Zaw Win Aung's hair was fairer when he was younger.

Figure 35 Another photograph of Maung Zaw Win Aung taken in December 1970. This photograph gives a closer view of Maung Zaw Win Aung's eyes. They were essentially of Caucasian form. U Tin Tut's eyes (Figure 34) were of Mongolian form.

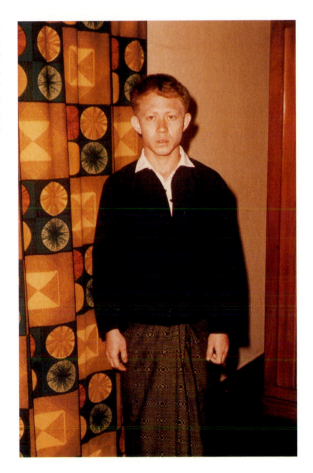

seats. Then we asked the proprietor whether he knew of any children who claimed to remember previous lives. A boy standing around heard us and immediately said that his younger brother was such a person. Thus we came to the case of Anurak Sithipan.

Anurak was born in Bangkok, Thailand, on December 14, 1969. At his birth he had a prominent birthmark of increased pigmentation near his right elbow (Figure 18). We met his parents and interviewed them and some other informants for the case. Anurak was believed to be the reincarnation of his older brother, Chatchewan, who had drowned about 3 years before Anurak's birth. The canals (called klongs) in that part of Thailand are tidal, sometimes dangerously so. Chatchewan had tied himself with a rope to a pier so that he would not be swept away with the current. It happened, however, that when the tide came in and the water rose, he was unable to detach himself from the rope, which held him under the rising water, and he drowned.

Before Chatchewan's body was cremated, a member of the family made a charcoal mark at his right elbow with the thought that when he was reborn he would be recognized by a birthmark at the same location. In most of the cases of experimental birthmarks that I have investigated the informants state that the birthmark was at exactly the location where the mark had been made on the dying or dead person. In Anurak's case, however, members of the family candidly stated that although both the charcoal marking and the birthmark had been at the right elbow, the charcoal marking had been farther forward than Anurak's birthmark was.

When Anurak became able to speak, he made a few statements referring to the life of Chatchewan. He spontaneously recognized and called by his nickname a young man known to Chatchewan. He searched for and found Chatchewan's boy scout uniform in a wardrobe that had other clothes in it. Anurak had a marked phobia of water.

Anurak's mother knew about the marking of Chatchewan's body, and we cannot summarily eliminate a maternal impression as a possible interpretation of his case. In the next case, that of Ma Choe Hnin Htet, a subject of Burma (born in Rangoon on September 27, 1976), we can exclude this interpretation. Ma Choe Hnin Htet's mother, Daw Myint Myint May, knew nothing about the marking of the body of Ma Lai Lai Way, of whom Ma Choe Hnin Htet was later thought to be the reincarnation. Ma Lai Lai Way had been the sister of Daw Myint Myint May.

Ma Lai Lai Way had congenital heart disease and was never healthy during her short life. Eventually, open heart surgery came to Rangoon, and Ma Lai Lai Way agreed to an operation that might modify, if not correct her congenital abnormality. Unfortunately, she did not survive the operation.

Three of Ma Lai Lai Way's schoolmates prepared her body for burial. They had heard of the belief that a mark placed on a dead person's body might generate a birthmark on a later-born baby; and they decided to test the belief by putting a mark of red lipstick at the back of Ma Lai Lai Way's neck. I interviewed all three of these persons independently and consider the testimony we have for the marking of Ma Lai Lai Way's body among the best we have for any such case. The young women did not tell members of Ma Lai Lai Way's family what they had done.

About 13 months after Ma Lai Lai Way's death, her sister, Daw Myint Myint May, gave birth to Ma Choe Hnin Htet. Soon after her birth Ma Choe Hnin Htet was found to have a prominent red birthmark at the back of her neck in the same location where Ma Lai Lai Way's schoolmates had marked *her* with lipstick (*). Ma Choe Hnin Htet also had a long birthmark, noticed much later, which was a thin line of diminished pigmentation that ran vertically from her lower chest to her upper abdomen (*). This corresponded to the surgical incision for the cardiac surgery during which Ma Lai Lai Way had died. I shall mention this second birthmark again in Chapter 12, where I discuss significant details of some of the birthmarks.

When Ma Choe Hnin Htet began to speak, she showed knowledge of Ma Lai Lai Way's life and in many ways tried to adopt Ma Lai Lai Way's position in the family. For example, she regarded her mother as her sister and her grandmother as her mother. She recognized some of Ma Lai Lai Way's friends, and I myself witnessed her correctly recognizing—without any guidance—one of them whom we brought to meet Ma Choe Hnin Htet for the first time.

Ma Choe Hnin Htet had no heart disease; she did, however, have a severe phobia of hospitals and anything to do with them, such as the taking of injections.

It happens that many children—perhaps one third of all children—are born with areas of redness at the back of the neck. In Western folklore this is often called a "stork's bite." The cause of these areas of redness is unknown. Most of them fade away as the child grows older, but the site is obviously not the best one for making experimental birthmarks.

I wish that persons marking bodies for experimental birthmarks would show more imagination than most of them do. The usual practice is to make a simple smudge, usually roundish, with some substance such as charcoal, and the related birthmark usually has a roundish shape that is not distinctive, particularly given that most nevi also tend to be roundish in shape.

In a few cases the markers have shown more originality. In a case in Burma, that of Maung Hla Win, for example, the mark was made (with grease from a cooking pot) around the sole of the foot of the child being marked. This is an uncommon site for nevi, and the resulting birthmark was also much larger than the usual nevus (Figure 19).

A similar large mark in an unusual place was made in the case of Ma Zin Mar Oo, another subject of Burma. The mark and the birthmark in her case were both wide, ran almost entirely around the lower leg, and were located just above the ankle, another infrequent site for nevi (*).

Dr. Jürgen Keil has investigated a case in Thailand in which the experimental birthmark looks as if someone had stroked the subject's arm with three separated fingers; and this appears to be what the person making the mark on the deceased person—a baby in this case—had done.

11

CHANGES IN THE APPEARANCE AND RELATIVE LOCATION OF BIRTHMARKS

In previous chapters I occasionally referred to birthmarks that had become fainter or had faded altogether as the subject grew older. For example, I mentioned in Chapter 6 that several of Necip Ünlütaşkıran's birthmarks that his mother had noticed soon after he was born were no longer visible when Necip was in his teens. And one of Nasruddin Shah's birthmarks had entirely faded by the end of his childhood. From following subjects over several or more years I have sometimes observed the fading of birthmarks before my eyes, so to speak; and we have sometimes documented this with successive photographs. I will describe three such cases in this chapter.

Govind Narain Mishra was born in Mainpuri, Uttar Pradesh, India, in August 1972. His parents were Brahmins, a fact relevant to the type of life that Govind Narain, when he could speak, claimed to have had.

When Govind Narain was about 3 years old, he began to refer to a previous life. He said that he had been a Dhobi (washerman) and that he had been bitten by a snake. This statement explained a prominent birthmark he had on the upper part of his right thigh, where the thigh joins the trunk at the pelvis. The birthmark was roundish; it had a pale central area surrounded by a ring of increased pigmentation. Govind Narain added some further particulars about the previous life, such as that he had had a wife who was fat and dark, two sons, and a daughter. He also said that he had owned three or four donkeys. (Many Indian washermen own donkeys, which they use to carry clothes to and from the rivers where they are washed.) One day he was sitting or crouching down and cropping grass for his donkeys when a snake bit him. As Govind Narain described how the snake had bitten him, he pointed to the site of his birthmark. Sometimes he would dream about the snake and, awakening, would say: "I was bitten by a snake."

In his play Govind Narain liked to go through the motions of washing and ironing; he wanted to wash the family clothes and eventually annoyed his mother by getting in her way as she did the washing. He had a marked phobia of snakes.

Govind Narain expressed a strong desire to find the wife of the previous life he was remembering, and he was sure that he could do so if taken to the area where he had previously lived. He implied, without specifically saying so, that he had lived elsewhere in Mainpuri. Unfortunately, he could state no proper names. On the other hand, washermen do not often die of snakebite, and Govind Narain's father thought that perhaps he could trace a person matching Govind Narain's statements. He took Govind Narain to the quarter of Mainpuri where the washermen lived and learned there about a washerman who had died of snakebite. His widow was said to have moved away. When Dr. Pasricha and I tried to follow this lead and verify the information for ourselves, however, we were unsuccessful, and I regard Govind Narain's case as unsolved.

During the several years when we followed the case (and those of two of Govind Narain's siblings who were also subjects of cases) we had ample opportunity to observe the fading of Govind Narain's birthmark. When we first examined it, he was 3 years old, and the birthmark was still prominent (*). Seven years later, when Govind Narain was 10½ years old, the birthmark had almost entirely faded. At the place where the birthmark had been I could barely discern a slight increase in the pigmentation of the skin compared with the surrounding skin (*). The area affected had also moved down somewhat as Govind Narain had grown.

Derek Betus was born in Gampaha, Sri Lanka, on January 22, 1979. He had a prominent birthmark—an area of decreased pigmentation—on his left great toe (*). When Derek began to speak about a previous life, he described that of a young boy, Maithripala, who had been bitten by a dog on the great toe of his left foot. The dog was probably rabid, and Maithripala seems to have died of rabies, although I never obtained a medical report of his illness, and the evidence from informants did not permit certitude in the matter.

Apart from some doubts about the cause of Maithripala's death, nearly all of Derek's statements were correct for his life. Derek also showed behavior appropriate for Maithripala.

During the period of investigating this case, which extended over several years, we had an opportunity to observe the fading of the birthmark on Derek's left great toe. By the time he was 7 years old it was no longer visible (*).

Faris Yuyucuer was born in Adana, Turkey, on August 24, 1970. At his birth he was found to have two birth defects and a birthmark. In this account I shall omit information about the birth defects and describe only the birthmark. It was an area of intense redness, round in shape, on his left buttock. It was about 1.5 centimeters in diameter (Figure 20). We saw and photographed Faris's birthmark when he was still an infant in arms—7 months old—and had not begun to speak.

On the basis of several announcing dreams Faris had already been identified as the reincarnation of a child of the neighborhood, Hasan Derin, who had drowned in July 1970 in a small lake not far from where he and also the Yuyucuer family lived. This boy had been burned on the left buttock when he was an infant, and a scar had remained there.

When Faris became able to speak, he talked about Hasan's drowning. He had a marked phobia of water and particularly warned other children not to go near the quarry where Hasan had drowned.

Later examinations of Faris's buttocks allowed us to observe how his birthmark faded. When he was 6½ years old, nothing of it remained, except perhaps a slight increase in pigmentation at the area where the birthmark had formerly been so prominent (Figure 21).

As I have shown, not all birthmarks fade as the subject becomes older. I believe that the majority of those I have examined have not faded. Why some birthmarks fade and others do not remains a matter for further research. In the ones that fade perhaps only the epidermis is affected, and the birthmark then heals like a first degree burn from which, as is well known, complete healing without a scar nearly always occurs. If the deeper layers of the skin are affected, either in a burn or a birthmark, a residue is likely to persist.

When a baby is born, its head comprises about one fifth of the total length of its body; but in a full-grown adult the head comprises only one eighth of the length (or height) of the body. This means that a marked change in the proportions of the various segments of the body occurs between birth and full growth.

Birthmarks frequently shift in position relative to anatomical sites as a child grows. In earlier chapters I have mentioned such shifting of the birthmarks in the cases of Chanai Choomalaiwong, Nasruddin Shah, Susan Wilson, and Susumu Ogura. I will describe one more example next.

Ravi Shankar Gupta was born in Kanauj, Uttar Pradesh, India, in July 1951. At his birth he had a large linear birthmark extending horizontally across the lower third of his neck. One observer described it as giving his head the appearance of having been glued on.

When Ravi Shankar became able to speak, he said that he had been the son of Jageshwar and had died from having his throat cut. These and other statements that Ravi Shankar made matched events in the short life of a boy called Munna, who was the son of Jageshwar Prasad. Munna's family lived in another quarter of Kanauj. Munna had been brutally murdered by having his throat cut in January 1951.

When I first met Ravi Shankar in 1964, he was a youth of 13. By this time the birthmark had migrated (and also faded) so that it consisted of a linear mark crossing his neck under the chin. It was then about 5 centimeters long and 4-5 millimeters wide. As Ravi Shankar continued to grow, the mark continued to shift upward. In 1971, when he was 20 years old, the birthmark was a line of increased pigmentation on the skin under his chin near its point (*).

As with the causes of the fading of birthmarks, we know little about why some birthmarks shift in relative position and others do not. It seems probable that the birthmarks most likely to shift in relative position are those in parts of the body most involved in relative changes in their proportions, such as the head, neck, and trunk. I do not remember having been told that any birthmark on an extremity changed in position as the subject grew. Govind Narain Mishra's birthmark may be an exception, but his birthmark was at the extreme upper end of his thigh. The birthmark of another subject (reported in the monograph, but not in this work) migrated, as the subject grew, from the lower part of the buttock to the upper thigh.

12

CORRESPONDENCES
OF DETAILS BETWEEN
BIRTHMARKS AND RELATED
WOUNDS OR OTHER MARKS
ON DECEASED PERSONS

Although the most important feature of the birthmarks that I describe in this work is their close correspondence in location to wounds (or other marks) on a deceased person, some of them have unusual details that seem to me scarcely less important than the correspondences in location.

I have already mentioned some of these correspondences of details. Four occurred in connection with surgical operations on the previous personalities. Muhittin Yılmaz had a horizontal, linear birthmark that had the location and appearance of the scar of a transverse incision for a surgical operation on the gall-bladder or nearby organs. Susumu Ogura had a crescentic birthmark behind his ear that had the shape of the standard surgical incision for mastoidectomy. Ma Choe Hnin Htet had a vertical, linear birthmark near the midline of her trunk that corresponded to the surgical incision for the open heart surgery that her aunt, whose life she remembered, had undergone. Juggi Lal's birthmark corresponded to a surgical opening of an abscess with subsequent stitching of the wound.

One of the most frequent of these important details occurs in the cases in which the subject has two birthmarks related to bullet (or shotgun) wounds of entry and exit. I have already described eight cases with this feature: those of Maung Sein Win, Henry Elkin, Chanai Choomalaiwong, Maung Tin Win, Metin Köybaşı, Tali Sowaid, Alan Gamble, and Cemil Fahrici.

I have investigated 14 cases of this kind myself, and my associates have investigated another 4, making a total of 18 such cases. These cases have the additional interest that in 14 of them one birthmark was larger than the other. The smaller birthmark was usually round or roundish and the larger one irregular in shape. In 1 of the 4 exceptional cases the bullet did not exit, in 2 of the cases the second birthmark had faded before I examined the subject, and in the fourth case the birthmarks were of about the same size. In several of the 14 cases with two birthmarks of different sizes, we could not learn which corresponded to the wound of entry and which to the wound of exit. There were 9 cases, however, in which the smaller birthmark corresponded to the wound of entry and the larger one to the wound of exit. This detail accords with the fact—well-known to forensic pathologists—that bullet wounds of exit are nearly always larger than wounds of entry. The difference results from the tendency of the bullet, in most cases, as it goes through the body to tumble and yaw and to push ahead of itself portions of bone or other tissue, thus producing a larger wound at the point of exit.

I will next describe some cases with other unusual details in the birthmarks.

Ma Mu Mu was born in Upper Burma on July 29, 1949. Her parents were U Aung Ba and Daw Nge Ma. Before Daw Nge Ma conceived Ma Mu Mu, U Aung Ba had a dream in which a deceased relative, Daw Ngwe Khin, appeared, sat on his knee, and said that she was coming to live with him and his wife.

When Ma Mu Mu was born, she was found to have two prominent birthmarks at the upper, inner part of her left breast. The two birthmarks were both round, but of different sizes, as can be seen in Figure 22. These birthmarks provided a further indication to Ma Mu Mu's parents that she was the reincarnation of Daw Ngwe Khin, because they knew how Daw Ngwe Khin had died.

A period of extreme lawlessness in Burma followed the defeat there of the Japanese Army by the British Army in the spring of 1945. The ensuing vacuum of authority encouraged local bandits to prey on the villagers. For their better protection many of the villagers withdrew into hutments outside the villages. During a period of unusual confusion, Daw Ngwe Khin, who had been outside her village in one of the hutments, decided to return to the village with some friends. As they approached the village, one of its defenders mistook them for attacking bandits and fired his shotgun at them. Daw Ngwe Khin was struck with pellets in the chest, and she died almost instantly, from a wound in her heart or in one of the nearby large blood vessels.

The significance of the two birthmarks of different sizes on Ma Mu Mu derives from the fact that the cartridge fired at her contained shot of different sizes. Although a reliable firsthand informant for the case told me this, I made extensive inquiries among manufacturers of shotgun cartridges with a view to learning whether they had manufactured cartridges with shot of different sizes. Two British manufacturers did not do this, but an American one later did, and it is possible that a manufacturer in India had produced such cartridges earlier. Also, in Burma owners of shotguns sometimes altered the pellets in the cartridges thus making what is called a "home load." My informant mentioned above had himself taken a shotshell apart and observed that it contained shot of different sizes.

Ma Mu Mu began to speak about the life of Daw Ngwe Khin when she was about 3 or perhaps 4 years old. She herself later did not remember having spoken about the previous life until an occasion when she was ill, between the ages of 6 and 7. She then had a remarkable upwelling of memories that were so intense that she seemed to be reliving parts of Daw Ngwe Khin's life.

Daw Ngwe Khin had adopted a baby girl, and she was carrying this child in her arms she was shot. Ma Mu Mu remembered that before Daw Ngwe Khin died she was able to ask the people around her to look after her child. Later, Ma Mu Mu became much attached to this girl, whom she regarded as her daughter. Like many subjects of these cases, Ma Mu Mu had a phobia—hers of firearms.

Obike Nwonye, an Igbo, was born in Obeagwu Ozalla, Anambra State, Nigeria, on January 7, 1973. He was born with a prominent birthmark roughly triangular in shape, on his right upper chest. By the time he was 11 years old, when I met and photographed him, the birthmark was approximately 2 centimeters long on each side. The surface of the birthmark had multiple small depressions, each approximately the size of a shotgun pellet (*).

Obike never spoke about a previous life. On the basis of his birthmark (with confirmation by an oracle) Obike was identified as the reincarnation of his great-grandfather, Nwachime, who had been killed during a tribal battle. He had received the discharge of a shotgun at close range and must have died almost instantly. He was thought to have died in about 1937.

I expressed some surprise that the location of Nwachime's wound would be remembered so precisely after so many years, but my informants were even more surprised at my puzzlement. For them, the wounds their relatives received in battle would be easily memorable. Obike's father told me that his father, Nwonye, had seen Nwachime's wound when he was a young boy of about 10; Nwonye had then lived long enough to see Obike's birthmark, which he said was at the site of Nwachime's wound.

Obike Nwonye is the fourth subject of this work with a birthmark corresponding to a wound from a shotgun; the other three are Hanumant Saxena (Chapter 6), Alan Gamble (Chapter 6), and Ma Mu Mu. Although the wounds were similar, the birthmarks were not, which permits me to repeat the point I made in Chapter 9: Wounds make poor predictors of the types of birthmarks to which they may later correspond.

Victor Vincent, a Tlingit, died in the spring of 1946 in Angoon, Alaska. He had been especially fond of his sister's daughter, Mrs. Corliss Chotkin, Sr. About a year before his death, he said to her: "I'm coming back as your next son. I hope I don't stutter then as much as I do now. Your son will have these scars." With that he pulled up his shirt and showed her a scar on the upper right side of his back. Then he pointed to a scar at the base of his nose near his right eye. As an additional reason for wishing to be reborn in the Chotkin family, Victor Vincent mentioned that he believed his deceased sister, Gertrude, had already been reborn as their daughter; and he liked the prospect of being again with his sister.

The scar on Victor Vincent's nose was the residue of an operation he had had to remove the right tear sac. I obtained a copy of the hospital report of this operation. I was not successful in obtaining a medical report relating to the scar on Victor Vincent's back. I did learn from one hospital, however, that he had been diagnosed there as having moderately advanced pulmonary tuberculosis of the upper part of his right lung. Although this particular record mentioned no operation, it is possible that at some other hospital Victor Vincent had had a biopsy or perhaps drainage of a pleural effusion or lung abscess.

About 18 months after Victor Vincent's death, Mrs. Chotkin gave birth to a son, Corliss, Jr. He was found to have two birthmarks at the locations Victor Vincent had predicted: one at the base of the nose (*) and one on his right upper back (*). The latter was particularly interesting, because alongside the main linear scarlike birthmark there were tiny punctate scars suggestive of the scars that are left after surgical stitches. Both of these birthmarks had migrated as Corliss grew. The one on his back moved downward. The one at the root of the nose had also moved downward, so that when Corliss was 15 years old this mark was actually on the lower part of the right side of his nose.

When Corliss, Jr. became able to speak, he made two statements about events in the life of Victor Vincent. He also spontaneously recognized some persons known to Victor Vincent.

Corliss, Jr. showed some behavior in which he resembled Victor Vincent. Victor Vincent had been left-handed, and Corliss was left-handed when he first began to write, but under pressure from a teacher he learned to write with his right hand. Like Victor Vincent, Corliss stuttered when he was a young child, but with the help of a speech therapist he overcame this defect. Victor Vincent had considerable mechanical skill, and Corliss when young showed a similar facility with engines, a capacity that he did not acquire from his father, who had no aptitude for engines.

Ma Win Win Nyunt was born in Rangoon, Burma, on March 27, 1957. Her case was complicated because her parents identified her as the reincarnation of her paternal grandmother and also believed that she had had an "intermediate life" as her own older brother. He was Maung Maung Ley, and he had been born and died between the death of Ma Win Win Nyunt's grandmother and her own birth.

He was 3 years old when he died. Ma Win Win Nyunt had no imaged memories of the life of Maung Maung Ley, and her identification as the reincarnation of him depended entirely on birthmarks. Some of these were experimental birthmarks that a servant had made on the body of Maung Maung Ley before he was buried. The servant had told no one that he had placed these marks, but when Ma Win Win Nyunt was born, he examined the baby and said that the birthmarks on her corresponded to the marks he had made on Maung Maung Ley.

I have included the case in this chapter not because of the experimental birthmarks, but because Ma Win Win Nyunt had another birthmark that was much more distinctive. Maung Maung Ley had died of leukemia, and during his last days he had been given intravenous injections through a needle placed in a vein at his ankle. The needle had been held in place by a strip of adhesive tape that was still attached when Maung Maung Ley died. Ma Win Win Nyunt had a birthmark of slightly increased pigmentation at the site of this adhesive tape, and it had the straight lines of the adhesive tape. I did not try to photograph it, but I did make a sketch of it (*).

Mehmet Karaytu was born in 1931 in the village of Kavaklı, near Adana, Turkey. He was born with a large triangular-shaped birthmark in his lower back (*). When he was about 3½ years old, he began to speak about the previous life of a man called Haydar Karadöl, who had been the owner of some farmland with a partner.

One day Haydar had been drinking and eating with his partner, when they began to quarrel. Haydar beat up his partner and then walked away. The man he had beaten, however, picked up a kitchen knife and, running after Haydar, thrust it into his back. Haydar died almost immediately. Mehmet remembered that he was still living when taken to a hospital, but I did not verify this detail.

Kitchen knives are single-edged, and the shape of Mehmet Karaytu's birthmark corresponded to the triangular profile that such a knife has.

Tong In Songcham was born in the village of Sao Lao in the province of Kalasin, Thailand, in May or June 1942. Immediately after Tong In's birth, her mother, Tam, noticed that she had a birthmark on her back that was bleeding. In fact, she had three birthmarks, but only one was bleeding. They were narrow linear areas of diminished pigmentation, all near the midline of her back. In Tong In's adulthood they were about 6-8 centimeters long and 3 millimeters wide (*).

Before Tam became pregnant with Tong In, her (Tam's) sister had a dream in which Tam and three other women, including the dreamer, were returning to their village when they met a woman who was standing alone. This woman approached and touched each of them to see which was cold. (In Thailand, a hot country, coolness of the body is considered a desirable quality.) Tam was the coolest, and so the woman—presumably a discarnate person—followed Tam to her home. This dream accorded with some statements that Tong In made when she began to speak about a previous life. She said that after dying she had walked from the village where she had died to Sao Lao. On the way she met four women and touched each of them. Tam was the coolest, and so she had followed her.

Tong In also described how she had died in the previous life. Her name had been See, and she had been married. One day her husband and his brother had a serious quarrel, and her husband, evidently fearing violence on the part of his brother, ran away. The brother was so angry that he seized an axe and attacked See. He chopped her three times in the back with the axe, and then put his foot on her and withdrew the axe. Tong In said that after dying she remained around See's house for a time and then began walking toward Sao Lao.

Tong In's statements about the previous life were correct for a woman called See, who had been killed, as Tong In described, in the village of Nong Khun Puwa, which is about 6-7 kilometers from Sao Lao. Tong In was born about a year after See's murder.

Tong In had no strong desire to return to Nong Khun Puwa, but eventually did so and there recognized a tree that See had planted.

I did not independently verify that See's brother-in-law had chopped *three* times with the axe when he killed her. Because Tong In's account of the murder tallied well with what I could verify about it—that See had been killed by her brother-in-law with an axe—I believe she was probably correct in this detail. If so, then the case includes a correspondence between three unusual birthmarks on the subject and corresponding wounds on the deceased person whose life she claimed to remember.

Charles Porter, a Tlingit, was born in Sitka, Alaska, in 1907. He was born with a prominent birthmark—an area of increased pigmentation—on his right flank, approximately over the right side of his liver. During his adulthood it was roughly diamond-shaped and measured about 4 centimeters in length and 1.5 centimeters in width (*).

When Charles Porter was a small boy, he used to say that he had been killed by a spear in a clan fight among the Tlingit. He named the man who had killed him, stated the place where he had been killed, and gave his own Tlingit name of the previous life. The man killed according to Charles Porter's description had been his mother's uncle.

When Charles Porter spoke about being killed with a spear, he pointed to his right side at the location of his birthmark. At this time, however, he was unaware that he had a birthmark there; because it was on the extreme of his flank, he might not have been able to see it easily.

By the time I investigated this case in the 1960s Charles Porter was in middle age, but I was fortunate in being able to interview his older sister, who confirmed what Charles Porter himself told me about his memories as a child. (He no longer had any imaged memories himself.) She remembered that he had been born with the birthmark on his flank. She said that he continued to talk about the previous life until he was about 8 years old. Their mother had tried to stop him from talking about it, perhaps because the man who had killed Charles Porter's great-uncle was still living, although he was by then an old man.

I was unable to learn when the clan fight in which the uncle had been killed had occurred. Clan fights among the Tlingit occurred frequently up to the last quarter of the 19th century, when they ceased. I suppose, therefore, that Charles Porter's uncle was killed not later than the early 1880s. Even so, the interval between his death and Charles Porter's birth would be long for cases among the Tlingit known to me.

Derek Pitnov, a Tlingit, was born in Wrangell, Alaska, in 1918. When he was born, he was found to have a prominent birthmark on his abdomen. It was located about 2 centimeters to the left of the umbilicus and slightly below it. The mark was diamond-shaped in form and in adulthood measured about 2 centimeters long and 1 centimeter wide. The birthmark had diminished pigmentation compared with the surrounding skin (*). There was a slight depression in the center of the birthmark. Derek Pitnov said that when he was a child and became cold, as after bathing in cold water, the birthmark would become deeper in color and take on the appearance of a recent wound.

On the basis of this birthmark and solely on its basis, Derek Pitnov was identified as the reincarnation of a celebrated Wrangell leader known as Chah-nik-kooh. He had been killed treacherously by the Sitkas when he had led a peace-making party from Wrangell to Sitka. He had died in 1852 or 1853.

Doubts might be expressed—I expressed them myself—about how informants could remember the exact location of a wound after more than 65 years. This is credible, however, to persons familiar with the accuracy of oral tradition among peoples like the Tlingit. Although most of the party of Wrangells were massacred by the Sitkas, a few survivors among the Wrangells reached home, and they recounted the bravery with which Chah-nik-kooh met his death as he became aware that the Sitkas were going to kill them. The location of his fatal wound would therefore be one of many details of the massacre that tribal members would transmit orally with exactitude.

Derek Pitnov never had any imaged memories of a previous life. He did have a marked phobia of bladed weapons that persisted into his adulthood.

The Tlingit battle spear seems to have had the conventional diamond shape of many spears (*), and I believe that the spears used to kill Charles Porter's great-uncle and Chah-nik-kooh were almost certainly of the same type. The birthmarks on Charles Porter and Derek Pitnov were both roughly diamond-shaped; and yet otherwise they were different in appearance, which suggests again the important role of the subject's skin in the processes producing a birthmark.

Ma Myint Myint Zaw was born in Pyawbwe, Upper Burma, on December 14, 1973. Her parents were U Kyaw Tint and Daw Mya Kyin. About a month after

Ma Myint Myint Zaw's birth, her mother noticed a round birthmark on the instep of her left foot. This observation made her think that Ma Myint Myint Zaw might be her deceased son reborn.

This son, Maung Pho Zaw, had been a boy of about 4 when he died under the following circumstances. He was playing with a top early one morning when he overheard his uncle, U Tha Hla, say that he was going to Myeinigone village. Maung Pho Zaw stopped playing with his top, picked it up, and followed his uncle, who took him by the hand. On the way, they crossed some fields, and Maung Pho Zaw suddenly cried out with pain. His uncle thought at first that Maung Pho Zaw had stuck himself with a thorn, but the boy pointed to a snake curled up nearby and then showed the instep of his left foot, where blood was oozing from a bite wound. (The snake was almost certainly a Russell's viper, a species of snake abounding in the fields of Burma.) It happened that some women were passing by just then, and one of them was smoking a cheroot. U Tha Hla took the cheroot from the woman and applied it to the site of Maung Pho Zaw's wound. He also put around the boy's leg a tourniquet that he made from the string of Maung Pho Zaw's top. U Tha Hla then hurriedly took Maung Pho Zaw to the nearest hospital. There the doctors rebuked U Tha Hla for burning Maung Pho Zaw's wound, which is a common but futile folk remedy for snakebite in Burma. The doctors themselves, however, could do nothing to save Maung Pho Zaw, and he died on the evening after he was bitten.

Maung Pho Zaw was the only son of his parents, and his death affected them greatly. About 2 or 3 months after Maung Pho Zaw's death, a neighbor of his family dreamed of seeing Maung Pho Zaw as a discarnate personality who said he was trying to find his way home, but did not know the way. At almost the same time, U Kyaw Tint dreamed that Maung Pho Zaw came to him and told him that he had come home. Soon after these dreams, Daw Mya Kyin became pregnant, and Ma Myint Myint Zaw was born about a year after Maung Pho Zaw's death.

When she became able to speak, Ma Myint Myint Zaw made only a few statements about the life of Maung Pho Zaw. She said that she was Pho Zaw and had been bitten by a snake. She pointed to her left foot to indicate where the snake had bitten Maung Pho Zaw. She made no statements outside the normal knowledge of her parents. When she was about 2 years old, Ma Myint Myint Zaw somehow found Maung Pho Zaw's clothes, pulled them out, and claimed them as hers.

Ma Myint Myint Zaw had a strong phobia of snakes, and this persisted at least up to the time of our investigation of the case, when she was 12 years old. She was then still afraid to go out of the house after dark for fear of not seeing a snake that might bite her.

Ma Myint Myint Zaw's most unusual trait, however, was her markedly masculine behavior. She first showed this at the age of 2, when her parents tried to get her to wear earrings, which she strongly resisted. They had to yield. This occurred at about the time she began to say that she was Maung Pho Zaw.

When Ma Myint Myint Zaw discovered Maung Pho Zaw's clothes—also at the age of about 2—she insisted on wearing them, and her parents allowed her to do so. After that she continued to wear boys' clothes almost exclusively. She showed other masculine traits also, such as a boyish gait.

When Ma Myint Myint Zaw reached school age, she went to school wearing boys' clothes and sat among the boys in their class at school. Her teachers overlooked this for some years, but in 1983—when Ma Myint Myint Zaw was about 9 years old—an inspector of schools did not. He discovered Ma Myint Myint Zaw sitting among the boys and expostulated. Ma Myint Myint Zaw's teacher called her in and told her that she must come to school dressed as a girl. Hearing this, Ma Myint Myint Zaw burst into tears. Her parents then intervened and asked the school authorities to be more flexible. A compromise was arranged according to which Ma Myint Myint Zaw would come to school on 2 days a week and show herself wearing girls' clothes. Nothing was said about the other days of the week. Ma Myint Myint Zaw did not adhere even to this bargain, and the school authorities tacitly overlooked her violation of the agreement. Ma Myint Myint Zaw continued to dress in boys' clothes and to show other masculine behavior until her middle teens. She began to menstruate at the age of 17, and when she was 18 she married. Subsequently she gave birth to two children. During these years her behavior became feminine; she adapted well to the roles of wife and mother. Dr. Jürgen Keil met her for a follow-up interview in early 1996. At that time he and his interpreter noticed only traces of residual masculine behavior.

Ma Myint Myint Zaw's parents indulged her wish to wear masculine clothes, and U Kyaw Tint even said that he might have encouraged this behavior, partly because he still wished to have a son, but mainly because he wanted to spare Ma Myint Myint Zaw from the terrible distress she experienced when forced to wear girls' clothes.

The birthmark on the instep of Ma Myint Myint Zaw's left foot was a round area of scarlike skin, slightly depressed below the surrounding skin. When she was a little more than 12 years old, the birthmark was about 1 centimeter in diameter (*).

Both U Tha Hla (who had applied the cheroot to Maung Pho Zaw's snakebite wound) and U Kyaw Tint confirmed to us the correspondence between the wound (from the snakebite and burn) on Maung Pho Zaw and the round birthmark on Ma Myint Myint Zaw.

Maung Htay Win was born in the village of Myaukthike, Upper Burma, on November 21, 1970. His parents were U Maung Pu and Daw Ma Gyi. Maung Htay Win was born with two narrow linear birthmarks on his left forefinger (*). When he was an adult, they were about 1 and 1.5 centimeters long and had diminished pigmentation compared with the surrounding skin.

These birthmarks did not lead to Maung Htay Win's being identified as the reincarnation of any deceased person. When he was about 4 years old, however, he said that he was called U Chit Saya, and he made a number of references to U Chit Saya's life and death. U Chit Saya had been U Maung Pu's stepfather, and he had died of snakebite.

U Chit Saya was a farmer who died when he was about 60 years old. On the day of his death he had finished work, and after tying up his oxen he had sat down on a pile of ground-nuts. He did not notice a snake that was nearby, and it bit him on the left forefinger. Someone sent for his son-in-law, U Chan Aye, and when U Chan Aye arrived he took a razor and cut the site of the snakebite. He then tried to suck out the venom, but U Chit Saya died the same night.

U Chan Aye later told U Win Maung (my assistant) that the birthmarks on Maung Htay Win corresponded to the cut (singular) that he had made on U Chit Saya's left forefinger before he sucked out the venom. It is not clear, therefore, whether he made only one cut or two cuts. He might have made just one, if he thought that the other wound was large enough to enable him to suck out the venom.

Maung Htay Win began speaking about a previous life when he was 4 years old. Watching his family's oxen being hitched up to their cart, he said: "Don't use these oxen. I have got mine." Asked to explain this remark he pointed to a cattle pen and then tried to find "his" oxen there. It did not occur to him that the oxen he was looking for had long since gone, but he correctly identified where they had been tied up. He also asked U Chit Saya's wife to return his (U Chit Saya's) clothes; and he asked for a crossbow that he said belonged to him.

When Maung Htay Win—still as a young child—met U Chan Aye, he held up his left forefinger and said it was the finger U Chan Aye had cut with his knife.

When Maung Htay Win was young, he showed the "adult attitude" that I mentioned in connection with the cases of Chanai Choomalaiwong, William George, Jr., and Ma Choe Hnin Htet. He addressed his father as "Maung Pu," which would have been appropriate for U Chit Saya, but not for a young son speaking to his father. In talking to one of U Chit Saya's sisters he addressed her with the junior honorific "Ma," instead of with the more respectful one, "Daw," which the Burmese use in talking to or referring to older women. As he grew older, however, he became more respectful to his elders.

Maung Naing was born in the village of Nyaunglunt, Upper Burma, on November 10, 1966. His parents were U Tha Gaung and Daw Kyi. Soon after Maung Naing's birth Daw Kyi noticed a birthmark on his left foot. There were actually two birthmarks, close together. They were linear, scarlike areas, slightly depressed below the surrounding skin and having slightly increased pigmentation. When Maung Naing was about 11½ years old, the birthmarks were about 1.5 centimeters long and 2 millimeters wide (*).

On the basis of a dream that Daw Kyi had and of Maung Naing's birthmarks, he was identified as the reincarnation of a deceased friend and next-door neighbor, Maung Tin, who had died of snakebite in 1965.

Maung Tin was a shopkeeper and inclined to be a heavy consumer of alcohol. One day the village policeman found him still at his shop after dark, and he advised Maung Tin to close up and go home; otherwise, the policeman said, he risked being bitten by a snake. Maung Tin replied somewhat rudely that the snake that would bite him had not yet been born. Nevertheless, he closed his shop and left for home. Within a few minutes, someone came running to tell the policeman that a snake had bitten Maung Tin.

The local dispensary had no antitoxin, and so Maung Tin was taken to a monastery 3 kilometers away, where the abbot was reputed to be skilled in treating snakebite. The abbot made two incisions at the site of the snakebite, but Maung Tin died a few days later. A villager, U Tin Maung, who had accompanied Maung Tin to the monastery and witnessed the abbot's incisions of the wounds, later told U Win Maung that Maung Naing's birthmark was at the site of the wounds on Maung Tin.

Maung Naing made a few statements about the life of Maung Tin. In particular, he said that he remembered that Maung Tin had been bitten by a snake on a moonlit night.

Maung Naing had a marked phobia of snakes. Maung Tin had had a tempestuous relationship with his wife, Daw Than, who was also a heavy drinker of alcohol. During one of their quarrels, she had openly wished that he would be bitten by a poisonous snake and die. As a child Maung Naing shunned Daw Than. He remembered how, in the previous life, she would get drunk and curse at him.

The important point regarding the last three cases is that the two birthmarks corresponding to wounds incised after snakebite were long and thin, whereas the birthmark corresponding to a snakebite wound that had been burned with a cheroot was round.

13

DISCREPANCIES BETWEEN BIRTHMARKS AND THE EVIDENCE OF REPORTEDLY CORRESPONDING WOUNDS

In previous chapters I have described only cases in which, if the case was solved, a correspondence occurred between the subject's birthmark and the wound (or other mark) on the concerned deceased person. In the great majority of the cases I learned of such a correspondence; but there were exceptions, and I will describe and discuss these in this chapter.

I had to select a measure of correspondence by which I would judge the closeness of the matching in location between birthmarks and wounds. I chose an area 10 centimeters square on a normal-sized adult body. Because the skin of such a body has a total area of 1.6 square meters, it would have 160 squares each 10 centimeters square. I chose this area because I thought it would allow both for some imprecision on the part of a pathologist who conducted a pertinent post-mortem examination and for possible failure on the part of adult informants to notice a shift in the position of a birthmark as the child grew (as I discussed in Chapter 11). A smaller allowed area might exclude some birthmarks for these reasons; but a larger one might wrongly include cases in which a discrepancy really had occurred. In many of the cases, such as those of Chanai Choomalaiwong, Alan Gamble, and Hanumant Saxena, the birthmark and corresponding wound were much closer in location than the area I selected.

My associates and I obtained altogether 62 documents bearing on the previous personalities' wounds and causes of death. Nearly all of these were medical documents, such as postmortem reports, hospital records, or doctor's notes; but a few were other printed sources. For 13 cases I decided that the document itself was inadequate or that the testimony for the case included nullifying ambiguities and inaccuracies, such as a failure to notice a claimed birthmark at the child's birth or soon afterward.

After the deduction of these 13 cases, 49 cases with adequate documents and satisfactory testimony about details of each case remained. Of these I judged the correspondence close (within the limit I defined) in 43 (88%) of the cases, but not so in the remaining 6 (12%) of the cases. In the monograph I give reports of all 6 of these cases, but in this synopsis I will summarize only 2 of them. Before coming to these 2 cases I will first describe 1 of the 13 cases that I set aside as containing doubtful information.

Vasantha Gunasekera was born at Polgahawela, Sri Lanka, on July 8, 1972. His parents were W. G. Gunasekera and his wife, Menike. Vasantha's father was a rice farmer. The family lived at Weligamuwa in the Kegalle District.

Vasantha's parents noticed no birthmarks on him at or soon after his birth. When he was about 2 years old, he began to speak about a previous life. He stated numerous details about the life and death of a boy who had been shot and killed in a nearby village. Vasantha gave the name of the village and numerous other details of the boy's life.

Vasantha's statements were correct for a boy named Shelton Weerasinghe, who had lived at a place called Kaddawattiya, which is about 3 kilometers from Weligamuwa. On April 9, 1971, Shelton (who was then about 7½ years old) had been in his family's house with his father and other persons when a group of men approached the house and without warning fired shots into the house. (The assailants appear to have been political rivals of the Weerasinghes, and they seem to have determined to settle accounts with the Weerasinghes at the time of the disruption caused by the insurgency in Sri Lanka in April 1971.) Shelton was hit by a bullet in the chest and died almost instantly.

The two families concerned in this case knew each other, and there might have been some casual acquaintance between them; but they belonged to different castes and had no social relationships.

Vasantha's family knew about Shelton's death, and they also knew that some of Vasantha's statements were correct for Shelton's life. W. G. Gunasekera, however, had no interest in verifying Vasantha's statements. Vasantha wanted to meet Shelton's family and sometimes begged his family with tears to take him to his "real mother and father," which he believed Shelton's parents were; but his father feared that a meeting might lead to Vasantha's developing divided loyalties between the two families.

Eventually, Shelton's older sister, who had heard about Vasantha's statements, came to Weligamuwa and met Vasantha. He recognized her without prompting, and the following day he also recognized Shelton's mother, when she came to Weligamuwa.

The informants differed about when the question of a birthmark on Vasantha first arose. He had been talking about the previous life for at least 2 years before anyone thought that he had a birthmark. One day his father expressed some skepticism about his claims, and Vasantha pointed toward his chest and said: "Here is proof." (These were not necessarily the exact words of a child of 4 or 5 years, but this is what he meant.) His parents then looked at his chest and identified a round mark of diminished pigmentation above his *right* nipple toward the midline (*). It was about 1.5 centimeters in diameter. On his *right* upper back Vasantha had another mark, irregular in shape, about 1 centimeter long and 6-7 millimeters wide. It was slightly depressed and puckered (*). It could have been the scar of a healed furuncle. Vasantha's family believed that the mark on the right side of his chest corresponded to the wound of entry on Shelton and the mark on the back to the wound of exit. Their opinion was strengthened by statements from Shelton's parents. Shelton's father remembered only that Shelton had been shot in the chest, but his mother thought the bullet had entered at the center of the chest.

The postmortem report on Shelton showed that the bullet that killed Shelton entered his chest on the *left* side near the nipple. It exited at the *left* back. On its way through the body it tore the heart and pericardium. Death "was caused by wounding the heart with a firearm."

I set this case aside because it violated the rule that a responsible informant must report having observed a mark claimed as a birthmark at or almost immediately after a baby's birth. I have not, however, adhered to the rule in a few cases in which I became convinced that the marks in question were not acquired postnatally and were therefore congenital. Vasantha's case, however, was not one of these exceptions.

As I mentioned, the mark on Vasantha's right upper back was probably the scar of a healed furuncle. I have no explanation for the roundish area of diminished pigmentation on his right upper chest.

Next I will describe two cases in which the birthmarks were noticed immediately after the subject's birth and did not correspond to wounds on the deceased person whose life the subject remembered.

Pappu Singh was born in his mother's village of Uduatnagar in the Barabanki District of Uttar Pradesh, India, on August 12, 1971. His parents were Shivmangal and Mithilesh Singh. They lived in the village of Kussaila, in the Unnao District of Uttar Pradesh. They belonged to the caste of Thakurs. Shivmangal was a peasant farmer living close to poverty.

When Pappu was a few days old, first his grandmother and then his mother noticed that he had a birthmark beneath his right nipple (*). They thought that he had "a third breast," and Shivmangal Singh agreed with them when he saw Pappu's birthmark.

Pappu started speaking between the ages of 1 and 2. When he was between 2 and 3, he began referring to details of a previous life. He said that his name was Lala Bhaiya and that he had a mill at a place called Atah. He pointed to his chest and said that he had been shot there. Hearing this, his parents thought his birthmark must have corresponded with the wound where he (in the previous life) had been shot. At about this time Pappu's grandmother took him with her on a journey that included passing through Atah. Pappu saw a mill there and said that it was "his." Farther along, at a place called Pawa, near Bidhnu Bazaar, Pappu said: "I was killed at Bidhnu Bazaar."

Pappu's statements corresponded to events in the life of a prominent resident of the area whose full name was Shivshanker Lal Tiwari, but who was generally known as Lala Bhaiya. He was a Brahmin zamindar (landowner and tax farmer). He had been murdered (in March 1969) while returning from the market at Bidhnu Bazaar. In those days, the 1960s, wealthy landowners like Lala Bhaiya aroused the animosity of land reformers. The quasi-communist group known as naxalites were suspected of murdering Lala Bhaiya, and indeed they later claimed responsibility for his death.

Shivmangal Singh was well acquainted with Lala Bhaiya and, like everyone else in the area, he had heard of Lala Bhaiya's murder. They had not been socially connected, however, because of membership in different castes and a wide separation of economic circumstances.

Pappu's family members credited him with having made 10 statements about the previous life before he met members of Lala Bhaiya's family. Eight of these were correct; one was slightly off in that Pappu said that he was killed while going to Bidhnu Bazaar when in fact Lala Bhaiya had been killed as he was on his way home from the bazaar. Pappu was also wrong in saying that he had been on a bicycle when he was killed. Lala Bhaiya usually did go to the market on a bicycle, but on the day of his murder he went on foot. At Atah, Pappu recognized several members of Lala Bhaiya's family.

Pappu showed an "adult attitude" toward other members of his family. He called his father "Shivmangal" instead of using the Hindi word for father, and he denied that Shivmangal was his father. He also had one trait that was unusual in his family: He was notably cleaner than Indian children of his age. (Brahmins are more fastidious about cleanliness than members of the lower castes in India.) He did not, however, exhibit any of the "Brahmin snobbery" that has characterized and sometimes made unpopular some subjects who, born in lower caste families, have remembered previous lives as Brahmins and never allowed other members of their families to forget this.

We come now to the postmortem report on Lala Bhaiya. This showed that he had been struck on the head with a bladed weapon, which had fractured his skull. And he had been shot with a shotgun, with the wound of entry on the *left* side of the chest below the left nipple. Some of the shot had passed through the chest and exited on the right side near the axilla.

From this we have to conclude that Pappu had no birthmark corresponding to wounds on Lala Bhaiya. His parents and grandmother who said that he had "a third breast" were probably correct, because his birthmark, under the right nipple, is in the area where auxiliary nipples sometimes occur.

When Pappu pointed to his chest as he said that he had been shot there, his pointing was probably inexact, if not vague. It was sufficient, however, to make members of his family again aware of the birthmark (auxiliary nipple), and they understandably but incorrectly identified it as corresponding to the fatal wound on Lala Bhaiya.

I cannot say why Pappu had no birthmark corresponding to Lala Bhaiya's wounds. Why some subjects have no birthmarks corresponding to wounds on a deceased person is as great a mystery as why some do have them.

Amitha Herath was born in Galgamuwa, Sri Lanka, on January 27, 1970. Within a few days of Amitha's birth, her mother, maternal grandmother, and maternal aunt all noticed a birthmark beneath the outside of her right ankle (*). They attached no significance to this birthmark until Amitha began to speak about a previous life.

She started her account of the previous life when she was under 2 years of age. She did not give a name for herself in the previous life, but she said that she had lived in a place called Nithalawa. She also gave the names of some members of the family. She described the home they lived in, which she compared with her (present) home, obviously considering the previous one superior. It had for example, a tiled roof instead of the thatched one of her family's house.

Amitha said that she had wanted to prepare a lunch for her (previous) father and had gone into the garden to pluck some plantains. A cobra had bit her on the foot. As Amitha spoke about being bitten by a snake, she indicated the place where the snake had bitten her—the outer side of her right foot, below the ankle. When Amitha pointed to the outer side of her right foot, members of her family identified the birthmark they had noticed earlier, but had not understood, as the site where the snake had bitten the person whose life Amitha was describing.

It was not difficult for Amitha's family to verify her statements. Nithalawa is only about 7 kilometers from where Amitha lived. The families already had some acquaintance, and Amitha's mother had been a classmate at school of the older brother, Guneratne, of the person about whom Amitha was obviously speaking.

This person was a young girl called Muthumenike, and she had died (in May 1968) precisely in the manner that Amitha described: bitten by a snake in her garden. The members of her family—with an exception I shall note—believed that the snake had bitten Muthumenike on the outside of the right foot under the ankle.

The exception came from Muthumenike's older brother, Guneratne, who said in 1976 that the snake had bitten her on the toes of the right foot. Later, he changed his opinion and concurred with other members of the family that the bite had been at the back of the foot under the ankle.

The death certificate, which was filled out 18 days after Muthumenike's death, included the following notation: "Died after a coma due to a poison by a cobra bite on the right foot near the little toe on the sole of the foot."

It is impossible to choose among possible explanations for the discrepancy between the site of the snakebite given on the death certificate and the site pointed to by Amitha and accepted by her family (on the basis both of what Amitha said and the birthmark) as the place where the snake had bitten Muthumenike. This was also the site remembered by members of Muthumenike's family, except for Guneratne in 1976.

One interpretation is that the birthmark noted on Amitha under her ankle had some irrelevant origin, but was incorrectly adopted by members of her family and then by Amitha herself as the site of the snakebite. Amitha might have had no birthmark on her toes or a small one that quickly faded.

It is also possible that the death certificate is wrong. The persons who do the work of Medical Examiners in Sri Lanka, known as "Inquirers into Sudden Deaths," are not trained in law or medicine. They are generally competent, but they are not infallible. In this case the Inquirer, who had gone to Muthumenike's home and examined her wound before he completed the death certificate, may not have examined Muthumenike's body carefully. He might have been influenced by Guneratne's belief (at that time) that the snake had bitten his sister near the toes. Later, Guneratne changed his opinion and fell into line with other members of Muthumenike's family. If, however, his first memory was incorrect and led to a false entry in the death certificate, we would have an explanation for the discrepancy, which, as I have continued to think about the case, has seemed to me increasingly likely to be the right one. Moreover, I learned from Guneratne that the Inquirer made no notes of his examination of Muthumenike while he was at the house. It is therefore quite possible that when, 18 days later, he filled out the death certificate, his memory failed him, and he misremembered the site of the snakebite wound on Muthumenike.

From the appraisal of the correspondences and discrepancies that the medical documents revealed, we may state a measure of the confidence we should have in the testimony of informants relying on their memories. As I mentioned earlier, without the medical documents we would have been misled in about 12% of the cases. In this 12% we would have incorrectly attributed a correspondence that did not exist. (In fact, the margin of error might have been somewhat less, because a study of errors made by informants showed that in four and possibly five cases, if we had relied on these persons' memories and had had no medical documents, we should have missed attributing a concordance that really did occur.) There is, therefore, some comfort in knowing that if we rely exclusively on the memories of informants, we will not go astray in more than one case in every seven or eight. Unfortunately, this would be a *general* rule and would say nothing about a *particular* case. We cannot know in advance in which case the informants' testimonies will be accurate and in which they will not. We have no substitute for medical documents in the study of the birthmarks in these cases; and we have not spared ourselves in trying to obtain them.

14

SOME CORRELATES OF BIRTHMARKS ATTRIBUTED TO PREVIOUS LIVES

The number of cases of children who claim to remember previous lives and who have relevant birthmarks seems sufficiently large to justify a search through the data for related features that would help us understand why some of the children have birthmarks and others who remember comparable deaths do not.

The first point to note is that the incidence of reported birthmarks varies widely between cultures. In a series of 895 cases from nine different cultures, 35% of the subjects had a birthmark (or birth defect); but the percentage of subjects with birthmarks (or birth defects) ranged between 6% for cases in Lebanon and 65% for those among the Igbo of Nigeria. In Chapter 1 I emphasized that our knowledge of the frequency of cases comes from *reported* cases; we have almost no understanding of the real incidence of cases. This is equally true of the cases with birthmarks. We know that some of the variance in cases with reported birthmarks derives from the greater attention given to them in some cultures than in others; birthmarks may occur just as frequently in India as they do in Nigeria, but they are not looked for as much in India as in Nigeria.

We can examine correlates of the birthmarks on the subject's side of the case, in events between the previous personality's death and the subject's birth, and on the side of the previous personality.

The subjects, as I have already emphasized, may contribute importantly by different reactivities of their skins. We know that skins, even of infants, react differently to irritants such as the toxin of poison ivy. It is reasonable to suppose therefore that they would also react differently to the mental influence of a discarnate personality that these cases suggest.

The birthmarks that correspond to wounds on a deceased person constitute a kind of physical memory of that person's wounds. It seemed important to ask, therefore, whether such a physical memory correlates with the abundance of imaged memories as expressed in the subject's statements about the previous life. I found no correlation. On the contrary, 21 subjects who had birthmarks and birth defects made no statements whatever about the previous personality with whom adults identified them on the basis of birthmarks, birth defects, or dreams. Another 7 subjects with birthmarks and birth defects made only one or two statements.

In most cases the subject was not conceived until months or years after the previous personality's death. There were numerous cases, however, in which the subject had been conceived before the previous personality's death. In a few cases with reasonably accurate testimony, the subject was born within a few weeks, or even days, of the previous personality's death. This would mean that the supposed mental influence was strong enough to modify a fetus already fully formed.

A small number of subjects claim to have had what I call "intermediate lives" between the previous personality's death and their birth. They sometimes make statements about such lives, but these are almost never verifiable. They may be fantasies. It is possible, however, that if such intermediate lives occur, an expected birthmark might appear on the body of the intermediate life but not on that of a later incarnation. I have, for example, studied in India two cases of subjects who claimed to have had intermediate lives after being murdered, one by shooting, the other by stabbing. Neither had a birthmark when one might otherwise have been expected. The cases with intermediate lives are too few to justify any conclusion. They perhaps give a hint, however, of a possible role of such lives as "erasers" of birthmarks.

As for the length of the interval between the previous personality's death and the subject's birth, I found no correlation between that length and the occurrence of birthmarks or birth defects.

This brings us to consider the condition of the previous personality at the time of death. I thought at one time that perhaps alcoholic intoxication might exert a protective effect against the occurrence of birthmarks and birth defects. I compiled a list of 14 subjects who remembered the lives of persons who were heavily intoxicated when they were killed. Of these 11 had birthmarks or birth defects and only 3 did not.

I would not, however, devalue the importance of further research concerning the relation of alcohol to birthmarks. The level of alcohol in the blood permissible

for drivers of vehicles must be legally fixed, usually at 100 milligrams per cen-
tiliter; but this is an arbitrary figure, and some persons may be intoxicated with
lower levels, whereas others are clinically sober with much higher ones.

The case of Maung Kyaw Thein of Pyawbwe, Upper Burma, illustrates the
difficulty of deciding the relevance of alcoholic intoxication to birthmarks. Maung
Kyaw Thein remembered the life of U Warzi, a well-known alcoholic who made
his living by selling paratas (a kind of pancake) in the town's market. He had enemies, and they decided to kill him. They waited until he shut up his little stall in
the market—it was about midnight—and waylaid him as he bicycled from the
market to his home. After cutting him up badly with sticks and knives, they left
him in a ditch. His son happened to pass by, heard his father's groans, and brought
him to a hospital, where he died a few days later.

Because U Warzi was a heavy regular drinker of alcohol, we can assume that
he had imbibed much during the day of his murder. On the other hand, he was sober
enough to ride his bicycle. Maung Kyaw Thein had verified imaged memories of the
life of U Warzi, but he had no trace of a birthmark corresponding to the knife cuts
that killed U Warzi. I am unable to say whether in this case alcohol might have
somehow inhibited one of the processes involved in the generation of birthmarks.

If alcohol does have a protective effect against birthmarks in these cases, the
effect might be due to whatever impairment of consciousness it induces.
Anesthesia would be another impairer of consciousness, but I have described
cases of surgical incisions (for example, those of Mehmet Yılmaz [Chapter 7] and
Ma Choe Hnin Htet [Chapter 10]), which must have been made while the previous
personality was under anesthesia, and to which birthmarks later corresponded.

Even so, we have evidence that some degree of consciousness is required in
the production of most birthmarks. (Experimental birthmarks are an obvious exception.) This evidence comes in the first instance from cases in which wounds were
more numerous than birthmarks. An example of this occurred in the case of Narong
Yensiri (Chapter 6). Another possible example occurred in the case of Nirankar
Bhatnagar (Chapter 4), although his statement that he was first hit on the head and
then stabbed remains unverified. It happens not infrequently in murders that the
assailants shoot, stab, or beat the victim repeatedly. If one of their early assaults produces loss of consciousness, say from a shot through the heart or a smashing blow
on the head, wounds inflicted after that event may not generate birthmarks.

The case of Ma Thoung illustrates as well as any known to me the role of
consciousness in birthmarks. Ma Thoung was born in the village of
Battakyaunggone in Upper Burma on November 5, 1945. When she was about 3
years old, she began to speak about a previous life as a person called Ma Mya

Sein, who had been executed by Japanese soldiers, earlier in 1945. Ma Mya Sein had been a trader who engaged in collecting and selling scrap iron. The occupying Japanese Army strictly forbade private trading in iron. It was such a profitable line of work, however, that Ma Mya Sein and some friends thought it worth the risk. Some Japanese soldiers caught them and decided to administer summary justice by beheading them on the spot. They lined up the group against a wall. Ma Thoung's memory of the last moment of Ma Mya Sein's life was that of a sword beginning to cut her neck. After that, she regained consciousness in the small body of Ma Thoung. The point of introducing this case here is that Ma Thoung had a birthmark with a slight defect at the lower tip of her left ear (*). Her case may be compared with that of Ravi Shankar Gupta (Chapter 11) whose birthmark extended (at the time of his birth) around the front of his neck, but not all the way round to the back. I believe that Munna, whose life Ravi Shankar remembered, retained consciousness while having his throat cut longer than did Ma Mya Sein as she was being beheaded. Maung Myint Aung's case (Chapter 4) is unverified, but it may be permissible to bring it into this discussion. After the Japanese soldier whose life he remembered had slit his throat, it would have taken him a minute or two to lose consciousness as he bled to death, and this may help us understand why Maung Myint Aung's birthmark extended right across the front of his neck.

The first shock in a fatal wounding may be influential in generating a birthmark. For example, in the cases of Sunita Khandelwal, Dellâl Beyaz, and Wilfred Meares (Chapter 6), a birthmark occurred at the point of impact where the heads of the persons whose lives they remembered hit the hard surface that stopped their falls; in these subjects, however, no obvious defect occurred at the site of injury that had caused the previous personality's death, such as a fractured neck or skull bone. In Alan Gamble's case (Chapter 6), his birthmarks corresponded to the place where the shotgun pellets went through the hand and wrist of Walter Wilson; he had no defect corresponding to the later amputation of Walter Wilson's forearm.

To conclude this chapter I will describe a case in which an injury after death corresponded to a birthmark.

Chamroon Kaochamnong was born in Tahrua, Thailand, on August 20, 1965. At his birth he was found to have an obvious birthmark at the top of his head. It was a roundish area of hairlessness, and when Chamroon was 9 years old it was about 1 centimeter in diameter (*).

On the basis of this birthmark Chamroon's father identified him as the reincarnation of a baby boy of the family who had died some 18 months before Chamroon's birth.

After the baby's death his father made a small coffin of wood in which he placed his dead baby son. He put the baby's body in this and carried it to the cemetery. When he arrived there, he noticed to his chagrin that he had somehow driven a nail through the end panel of the coffin at the baby's head so that it had wounded the baby there. He was convinced that the birthmark on Chamroon corresponded to the wound that he had inadvertently made on his dead baby's head.

Other examples of birthmarks and birth defects seemingly derived from marks and wounds made after death occur in the cases of experimental birthmarks (Chapter 10) and birth defects. (I describe experimental birth defects in Chapter 20.)

15

THE INTERPRETATIONS OF BIRTHMARKS RELATED TO PREVIOUS LIVES

Although some of the subjects whose cases I shall present in later parts of this book have birthmarks (as well as birth defects), I have now presented all the cases in which birthmarks (as opposed to birth defects) have been the subject's principal physical abnormality. It seems appropriate, therefore, to consider at this stage the several interpretations available for understanding these cases. By *understanding* I mean the endeavor to link the phenomena with branches of better established knowledge or, if need be, to judge them to be as yet outside such knowledge, for which we use the word *paranormal*.

Before we can consider alternative interpretations for the cases, we must decide that the reports we have are authentic. By *authentic* I mean that the reports given to investigators by informants and then set out by myself describe events with satisfactory closeness to the events as they really happened. This is the century-old endeavor of all investigators of spontaneous phenomena that appear to occur paranormally. It is, in principle, no different from the striving of lawyers to reconstruct the events of a crime or that of historians to understand what really happened in the past, *wie es eigentlich gewesen ist* ("what really happened"), as von Ranke said. No matter how much we try, we cannot know exactly what really happened, but that does not matter. What does matter is whether what we now believe happened approximates *sufficiently* to what did happen. Some critics believe that mistakes and discrepancies about details betray more serious flaws that should discredit any case in which they occur, which would be most of them. I do not believe this myself; but this is a matter readers should judge for themselves, and this gives me another opportunity to exhort my readers to study the details I have included in the monograph. For myself I will say that I believe all the cases included in the monograph and here are authentic by the definition I have given.

In recent years the independent investigations of colleagues have increased my confidence in the authenticity of the cases of the children who claim to remember previous lives. Four of them have replicated my investigations and have come, in general, to conclusions about the authenticity of the cases similar to mine. To be sure, they studied cases different from mine, and their investigations do not directly support my accounts of the cases I am here reporting. Because they followed my methods, however, albeit with their own modifications of details, their research encourages me to believe in the authenticity of the cases I have studied myself. I emphasize that the word *authenticity* refers only to the accuracy of the informants' descriptions of events and says nothing about the interpretation or explanation of those events.

Turning now to the interpretations of the cases, I will first discuss normal ones and then paranormal ones. According to the principal normal interpretation, the birthmarks we are trying to understand are not fundamentally different from the "ordinary" nevi and moles that everyone has, and their correspondence with wounds on a deceased person just occurs by chance. As for the statements and unusual behavior that informants attribute to the child, these, according to the view I am here describing, are either invented altogether by the subjects to account for the birthmark or they are imposed by the parents on the child, who learns to repeat what they expect it to say. The full phrase for this interpretation thus becomes "chance and fantasy," or, if we find or reasonably suspect that the subject's parents have imposed an identification on it, we can speak of "chance and suggestion."

Anyone considering this interpretation must admit that some of the birthmarks are indistinguishable from ordinary nevi, and I have described a few that are; but most of them are not. Instead, they differ from ordinary nevi in various ways that I have already mentioned, and the photographs of most of them clearly support my claim concerning this difference. Even so, the argument for a chance correspondence might apply to cases of single birthmarks corresponding to single wounds. As I mentioned in Chapter 13, the skin of a normal-sized adult would comprise 160 squares each 10 centimeters square. We can see that the odds against chance of a single birthmark corresponding in location with a single wound would therefore be only 1/160. When we consider the cases of correspondences between two birthmarks and two wounds, the odds against chance immediately increase and become 1/160 x 1/160, or (approximately) 1/25,000. There are, in fact, many cases in our series with two or more birthmarks. Moreover, many of these (and other) birthmarks have unusual details in which they correspond to details of a relevant wound. Although we cannot give a quantifiable weight to the likelihood of such correspondences of details, by some amount this feature (for the cases in which it occurs) further diminishes the likelihood of a correspondence occurring by chance.

As for the invention or imposition on the child of a fiction intended to explain the birthmark, I have already said that although this may sometimes occur, many parents and other informants—perhaps most of them—regard the child's statements and related behavior with indifference or positive opposition. They do not have a motive, let alone the time, for imposing an altered identity on a child. In Chapter 1 I mentioned that 41% of Indian parents had suppressed their children from speaking about a previous life. I do not mean to say that parents may not occasionally guide and even prompt a child in a direction of their own thinking, and I have already mentioned the risk of this when parents are prepared by dreams and birthmarks to believe that some deceased friend or member of the family has been reborn in their family. We should ask, however, how pliable children are to parental influences. The extent to which adults may influence a child to assume an identity that it would not otherwise adopt is perhaps amenable to scientific inquiry; and I welcome the endeavors of colleagues like Dr. Erlendur Haraldsson, whose studies with psychological tests of children in Sri Lanka who claim to remember previous lives indicate that they are not more suggestible than their peers.

Although dreams and birthmarks may prepare the way for the false elaboration of some cases, we can exclude this possibility in the numerous cases in which the two families live a considerable distance apart and when the evidence justifies our believing the informants who say that the families had no contact or knowledge of each other before the case developed.

If we set aside interpretations of the cases along normal lines, we need next to try to choose the best of several explanations that invoke some paranormal process.

The simplest of these explanations supposes that the subject of the case acquires through some kind of extrasensory perception all the information about a deceased person that he or she expresses in statements about a previous life. The subject would presumably be somehow tapping the minds of living persons who, from having known the concerned deceased person, would have the information that the subject would need to obtain. In cultures with a strong belief in reincarnation, from which most of these cases are reported, the belief would help to mold the information into the form of a supposed previous life. This interpretation has important weaknesses. First, with rare exceptions, the subjects provide no evidence of paranormal powers outside the claimed memories of a previous life, and none of them show any capacity for paranormal communication of the magnitude we should have to imagine if they are obtaining their information in this way. Second, the cases include much more than the cognitive details of mental images expressed in the child's verbal statements. Nearly all the children show a strong identification with the concerned deceased person and behavior that is unusual in their families but appropriate for that person. How does this happen? One must suppose the collaboration of the child's parents in shaping its personality to match that of the deceased person. I have said that this may indeed occur when the parents knew the person in question, but it could not happen when he or she was someone unknown to them. Or are we to suppose also that the parents as well as the child have unusual paranormal powers? Third, this interpretation fails to account for the birthmarks and birth defects that about one third of the subjects have.

A second paranormal explanation sometimes advanced for these cases attributes them to "possession" of the child by a discarnate personality. The latter is conceived as imposing its memories on the subject along with its likes, dislikes, and other behavioral characteristics. I am far from believing that something like possession cannot occur. Indeed, I have investigated cases with anomalous dates in which the subject has had memories of a person who was still living when the subject was born. I have published reports of three such cases and expect to publish reports of several more in the future. In these cases a recently deceased personality seems to take over or possess a body that was that of another living person. One weakness of the concept of possession as applied to the cases with birthmarks is its failure to account for the birthmarks. They, by definition, must be present at birth, which means that the discarnate personality must begin its influence on the subject while it is still a gestating embryo or fetus. If this happens, however, what is the difference between possession and reincarnation? A further weakness of the concept of possession applied to these cases is its failure to explain the almost invariable fading of memories that affects the subjects between the ages of 5 and 8. Why should a possessing personality, having successfully imposed itself on a child for some years, cease to do so? And why should all such possessing personalities cease their possessing at about the same period of the children's lives?

A third paranormal interpretation of the cases can at least account for the birthmarks. I refer to maternal impressions. I have already emphasized the importance of this interpretation for many cases, because the subject's mother in those cases had seen or at least learned about the wounds on the concerned deceased person. There are, nevertheless, 25 cases for which I am confident that the subject's mother had no knowledge of the previous personality's wounds. The interpretation of maternal impressions has the further weakness that it supposes that the mother of the child imposes on it, or imagines for it, all the statements and unusual behavior the informants attribute to it. This suggestion encounters the objection I mentioned earlier in connection with the normal interpretation of the cases: the lack of motive on the part of the mother (or father) to impose an identification of their choosing on the subject and the lack of evidence that they could succeed if they tried.

I accept reincarnation as the best explanation for a case only after I have excluded all others—normal and paranormal. I conclude, however, that all the other interpretations may apply to a few cases, but to no more than a few. I believe, therefore, that reincarnation is the best explanation for the stronger cases, by which I mean those in which the two families were unacquainted before the case developed. It may well be the best explanation for many other cases also. Yet in saying that I think reincarnation is the best explanation for many cases, I do not claim that it is the *only* explanation. Further research may show that it is not even the best one.

This is a matter about which my opinion should count for little. I regard my contribution as that of presenting the evidence as clearly as I can. Each reader should study the evidence carefully—preferably in the monograph—and then reach his or her own conclusion.

16

INTRODUCTION TO CASES WITH BIRTH DEFECTS

In previous chapters I have sometimes mentioned abnormalities that we could call birth defects. Examples occurred in the asymmetry of the breasts of Daw Aye Than (Chapter 5) and in the slight malformation of Ma Thoung's left ear (Chapter 14). In the following chapters, however, we pass from such minor defects to major ones, usually involving partial or complete absence of fingers, toes, and larger parts of arms, legs, ears, or other organs.

Apart from the gravity of such defects, they are much less easily attributed to chance than are birthmarks of which, as I mentioned earlier, almost everyone has one or more. In contrast to birthmarks, serious birth defects are comparatively rare.

The incidence of birth defects in the general population reported in different series varies between 0.74% and 3.30%. This somewhat wide range occurred partly because some of the series were of registered births, others of hospital births. Also, criteria for including particular defects varied as did the thoroughness with which the babies were examined. The best overall estimate of the incidence of birth defects is about 2% of births.

Several reports of surveys of birth defects have included information about the causes of the birth defects. Only a few causes of birth defects are definitely known. These are a) genetic factors, under which we may subsume chromosomal abnormalities; b) teratogens, such as certain infectious diseases and certain drugs and other toxins; and c) uterine conditions, such as the crowding during twin pregnancies. When we exclude these known causes, a large number of birth defects remain assigned to the category of "unknown cause." Reports of several series have offered estimates (or actual counts) of the cases with "unknown cause" ranging from 43.2% to as high as 70%.

Even the birth defects of known causation show a wide variation in the individual manifestations of the defect or defects usually associated with the identified agent. Experts have been forced to acknowledge that a single cause is rarely sufficient to produce a birth defect, and instead they allow for the interplay of several factors, called in medical terminology "multifactorial etiology." The principal claim presented here is that the influence of a reincarnating personality may be one factor we should consider in the causation of some birth defects.

I will next give several examples of birth defects that show the insufficiency of the idea of a single cause of some diseases for which one significant cause has been identified.

A simple example of multifactorial etiology occurs in the fairly common condition of cleft lip and palate. A wide range of abnormalities under this heading occurs. There may be only a slight "nick" in the lip or a whole range of severe divisions of the lip with and without cleavage of the palate. Cleft lip and palate appear to have an important genetic component. If one twin of a fraternal (dizygotic) pair has the condition, the other twin will be affected in 8% of cases; but in identical (monozygotic) twins, if one twin has the condition, the other has it in 38% of cases. Yet the significant point here is that in such twins, of identical genetic constitution and nearly the same uterine environment, 62% of the babies are *not* concordant for the condition. There have even been cases of conjoined (so-called Siamese) twins discordant for cleft lip. One study showed that psychological stress to the mother was a contributing factor in the causation of cleft lip, although a second study did not confirm this.

Marfan syndrome is a disorder of the connective tissue that produces a wide variety of defects throughout the body, but particularly in the eyes, heart and blood vessels, and bones. There are good grounds from studies of pedigrees for believing that a necessary cause of the condition is a single dominant gene, which some geneticists have reported locating on chromosome 15. Yet this gene may not be a sufficient cause. The clinical manifestations of Marfan syndrome vary so greatly that we have to suppose some other causative factor or factors besides the genetic component. Some affected persons will have symptoms predominantly in the skeletal system without ocular or cardiac symptoms. Other patients may have skeletal and ocular changes without cardiac lesions. These wide variations may occur in members of the same affected family. Geneticists use the term *variable expressivity* to account for these variations. This, however, is simply stating the obvious. "Modifier genes" are conjectured as variably influencing the expressivity, but they are rarely specified.

The condition known as polydactyly, in which a person affected has an extra finger or toe, also has an important genetic component. It too, however, exhibits a wide variety of manifestations in the individual members of an affected family. Here again, geneticists have introduced the concept of modifier genes in order to account for these variations.

German measles (rubella) in a pregnant woman appears to be an important causative factor in the occurrence of birth defects, notably in the eyes, ears, and heart. It is particularly damaging when the mother-to-be contracts the disease during the early weeks of her pregnancy. Yet in one series only 16.7% and in another only 15% of babies thus exposed were found to have major birth defects. Moreover, a puzzling one-sidedness of the effects may occur; one eye of a baby may be seriously affected, while the other one is normal.

Similar observations were made during the brief epidemic of malformations attributed to the drug thalidomide. Although there can be no doubt about its damaging effects, as many as 50% of the women who took thalidomide during a pregnancy delivered normal babies. Dosage and severity of the birth defects seemed unrelated. In studies of twins it was found that both were usually affected, but one twin might be much more affected than another. One case occurred in which one twin had hands attached to shoulders without any intermediate arms (phocomelia), and the other twin had normal limbs.

My drawing attention to the insufficiency of single known causes as the explanation for birth defects does nothing to support the explanatory value of previous lives as an additional factor. I have reviewed the importance of acknowledging multiple factors in the causation of birth defects only to weaken the widespread idea that present lines of inquiry will in time suffice to explain all we need to know. Doubt about the adequacy of present knowledge may stimulate interest in other lines of investigation, such as the one described in this book.

Instances of a disorder known as the constriction ring syndrome will be found among the cases of the following chapters. In this condition, a ring or band of tissue forms around a limb or a digit of a fetus. At the site of the ring the organ affected is constricted, and beyond the constriction there is often a swelling. Occasionally, the end portion of a fetal limb may become completely severed from the remainder of the body.

One theory to explain the constriction ring syndrome attributes the rings to amniotic bands of the gestational sac that become loose and then entangle and constrict the limbs affected. Amniotic bands, however, fail to account for all the features of some cases, especially cases of identical (monozygotic) twins having a common amnion with one twin affected and the other not.

A second theory of the constriction ring syndrome attributes the condition to a failure of development of the embryonic tissue beneath the skin at the site affected. The appearance of a constricting band is, on this view, illusory; the abnormality is one of failure of embryonic development. This theory has weaknesses also, especially if it is linked to hypothetical genetic factors, because there is no evidence of a genetic component in the condition. The cases of the present work showing the constriction ring syndrome suggest that the mental force in play, if I may use that expression, inhibits embryonic development at the sites affected, which appear to correspond to wounds in a previous life.

The birth defects that I describe in the following chapters are often of types unknown to experts on birth defects. They do not correspond to any commonly recognized syndromes of malformations. Others, however, do conform to those types. The monograph includes, for example, two cases whose subjects had a cleft lip, and I summarize one of these in Chapter 18 of this book.

In later chapters I occasionally describe birth defects of a known type as common or fairly common, rare, or extremely rare. Figures of the incidence of such birth defects in the general population are available, and I give them in the monograph. In the present work I shall use the descriptive terms without giving the precise figures of incidence. Readers should consider the rareness of a birth defect in appraising the likelihood that it might have corresponded to a wound on a deceased person by chance.

17

BIRTH DEFECTS OF THE EXTREMITIES

In presenting the cases with birth defects I have divided them into three groups: those in which a birth defect occurred in one or more of the extremities, those in which a birth defect occurred in the region of the head and neck, and those in which birth defects occurred in two or more regions of the body.

This chapter in the monograph includes 23 cases of which more than half are from Burma; and in most of the Burmese cases the previous personality was murdered, often with preceding torture. I will present summaries of only 7 of these 23 cases.

Lekh Pal Jatav was born in December 1971 in the village of Nagla Devi in the Mainpuri District of Uttar Pradesh, India. Lekh Pal was born without the fingers (phalanges) of his right hand, which were represented by mere stubs; his left hand was normal (Figure 23).

As an infant Lekh Pal was exceedingly frail, and his development in walking and talking was far behind that of his peers. He had just begun to talk and had spoken only a few words about a previous life when a woman from the village of Nagla Tal—about 8 kilometers from Nagla Devi—came to Nagla Devi and happened to notice Lekh Pal in his mother's arms. She mentioned that a child of Nagla Tal had had his fingers cut off in an accident. She, and perhaps some other villagers, took back information about Lekh Pal to the village of Nagla Tal.

In Nagla Tal a child called Hukum Singh had had his fingers cut off when he inadvertently put them into the blades of a fodder-chopping machine, which his father was operating without noticing that his little son, who was about 3½ years old, had approached the machine. Hukum Singh survived this accident, but he died the following year of some unrelated illness.

Hukum Singh's family seemed in no hurry to meet Lekh Pal, and before they had done so he had spoken to his family about the life of Hukum. He kept repeating the word "Tal, Tal," but at the time this made no sense to his mother. He said Nagla Devi was not his home and he would not stay there. His older sister later remembered that he described to her how, in the previous life, he had put his hand into a fodder-chopping machine. He said that he had a mother and father in "Tal" and also an older sister and a younger brother. He did not give Hukum's name. He indirectly identified Hukum's father as the person operating the fodder-chopping machine when his fingers were cut off.

Eventually a villager from Nagla Tal who had learned about Lekh Pal came over to Nagla Devi and took him to Nagla Tal, where he was credited with making a number of recognitions. For example, he pointed to the place where the fodder-chopping machine that cut off Hukum's fingers had stood; it is doubtful, however, whether he recognized the actual machine involved.

The two families concerned in this case lived in villages that might be considered close by Western readers; but if they take account of the limited means of transportation in the part of India where the case occurred, they can believe the informants' statements that the families had not known each other before it developed. It is true that there had been some exchanges, including at least one marriage, between the two villages; but I am satisfied that no one from Nagla Tal gave normal information to Lekh Pal's family about Hukum's accident before he spoke about it.

Lekh Pal's birth defect is extremely rare. A condition known as brachydactyly, which means "shortened fingers," occurs as an inherited trait in some families. In brachydactyly, the fingers are abnormally short; but they are present, not mere stubs, as were the fingers of Lekh Pal's right hand. Moreover, one-sided brachydactyly is an even rarer condition than the bilateral defect. In the monograph (but not in this book) I report one other case of unilateral brachydactyly.

An important detail for the later discussion of processes in these cases is the firm insistence by Hukum's family that his thumb had not been cut off when the other four fingers of his right hand were. Yet Lekh Pal's thumb was as much affected in his birth defect as the other fingers of his right hand. This permits me to introduce the concept of a psychical field as part of the process in the occurrence of some of the birth defects I describe.

Ma Myint Thein was born in the village of Okingone near Pyawbwe, Upper Burma, on October 12, 1956. Her parents were U Pe Tin and his wife, Daw Khin Hla. Before Daw Khin Hla became pregnant with Ma Myint Thein, U Pe Tin dreamed that an acquaintance, U Sein Maung, said that he wished to be reborn in

U Pe Tin's family. When U Pe Tin had this dream, he did not know that U Sein Maung was dead. The next day, however, he learned that assassins armed with swords had killed U Sein Maung the day before. It happened that on that day U Sein Maung had bicycled out from Pyawbwe to visit his parents. On the way back he had stopped and chatted a little with U Pe Tin and Daw Khin Hla before getting on his bicycle again and continuing on his way. He was waylaid by the murderers on the road back to Pyawbwe.

U Sein Maung had owned a truck with which he traded successfully between Pyawbwe and Rangoon. His frequent absences, however, had strained his marriage, and it was not improved when his wife learned that he had a mistress, or, as they say in Burma, a "lesser wife," in Rangoon. In a fit of despondency U Sein Maung's wife killed herself by drinking battery acid.

U Sein Maung was not murdered until 4 or 5 years after his wife's death. Robbery was not a motive, because the murderers did not take his bicycle and the jewels that he had been wearing. It was widely suspected that U Sein Maung's mother-in-law, Daw Saw Yin, nourishing vengeful thoughts about her daughter's mistreatment at his hands, had hired professional killers to murder him.

We were able to talk with two persons who had gone to see U Sein Maung's body after he was attacked and killed. (The murderers had left the body where they had killed him.) They said that the fingers of both of U Sein Maung's hands had been chopped off (by a sword) and his head almost severed from his trunk. An associate of mine, U Nu, who had not himself seen the body, made inquiries about the murder a few days after it occurred, and he said that the statements of the persons with whom he talked agreed with those of our later informants, although U Nu's informants mentioned that U Sein Maung had also been stabbed in the back.

Figure 24 shows Ma Myint Thein's hands as they appeared when she was 20 years old. All the fingers were markedly shortened and malformed, and most had constriction rings, such as I mentioned in Chapter 16. Only the left thumb was entirely normal.

Although Ma Myint Thein began to speak coherently when she was not more than 2 years old, she did not refer to a previous life until she was about 5, considerably older than most subjects of these cases when they begin to speak about a previous life. Many years later, Ma Myint Thein remembered that her first memories of the previous life occurred when, as she was playing with other children, she noticed that her hands were different from theirs. She then began to recall that in a previous life she had been murdered by three or four men with swords. Daw Khin Hla said that she first learned about Ma Myint Thein's memories when she overheard her saying to one of her older brothers: "I have got a wife in the south [meaning Rangoon]. I will give you candies if you will take me there."

After this, Ma Myint Thein gradually opened up her memories to other members of her family. She said that she had been called Sein Maung. She had a wife, Ma Thein, and two children, a boy and a girl. She gave other particulars that were correct for U Sein Maung, but I will pass over most of them in order to describe what she said about U Sein Maung's death.

She described how she had been killed with "a big long knife." (She used the Burmese word *dah*, which can mean any bladed instrument from a kitchen knife to a sword.) She said that her fingers were malformed because she had held up her hands to ward off the first stroke of the sword as the murderers began to attack U Sein Maung. She remembered later that U Sein Maung had been wearing a ring, a wristwatch, and a gold bracelet. (These would have been among the last objects in U Sein Maung's visual field when he held up his hands as he was being attacked.)

Ma Myint Thein had a phobia of the site where U Sein Maung had been killed, and when she had to pass it on her way to Pyawbwe, she found herself shivering. The malformation of her fingers distressed Ma Myint Thein greatly when she was young, and she sometimes tried to hide them.

Ma Myint Thein was convinced that U Sein Maung's mother-in-law, Daw Saw Yin, had contracted for his murder, and, not surprisingly, her relations with Daw Saw Yin were not cordial.

When she was young, Ma Myint Thein also showed masculine traits. She was fond of wearing boys' clothes and sometimes used the masculine verbs when speaking. (Like some other languages Burmese has some different word forms according to the speaker's sex.) She complained about being a girl.

As she grew older, Ma Myint Thein became better adjusted to her condition. In her early 20s she married and later had two normal children.

Ma Khin Mar Htoo was born in Tatkon, Upper Burma, on July 26, 1967. Her parents were U Thein Myine and Daw Ngwe Kyi. Before she conceived Ma Khin Mar Htoo, Daw Ngwe Kyi dreamed that a girl called Ma Thein Nwe was going to be reborn as her daughter. Ma Thein Nwe, who was nicknamed Kalamagyi (which means "big dark girl" in Burmese) because she was somewhat dark-complexioned, had died under the following circumstance in August 1966.

The trains in Burma had then no restaurant cars or vendors moving through the train to sell food and drinks to the passengers. Accordingly, at station stops vendors surrounded the trains and offered food, water, flowers, and other items for the passengers to buy. Kalamagyi and her mother earned a living selling to the train passengers in this way. The trains at Tatkon stopped on side lines beside the two platforms. There was a middle line between the two outside lines, and express trains not halting at Tatkon would pass through the station on that line.

On the day of her death, Kalamagyi was walking on the central line, confidently expecting the train to be switched onto the line next to the platform. She had flowers that she hoped to sell to the passengers and was walking along the line with her back to the engine. On that day, however, a switch failed to function properly, and the train, instead of moving to the side line beside the platform, continued on the central line. Horrified, the switchman saw that it would run down Kalamagyi. So did the engine driver who sounded his horn and braked the train. He was too late, and the train ran over Kalamagyi.

It was possible to some extent to reconstruct how Kalamagyi died under the train. Her lower right leg was found at a considerable distance behind the rest of her body, which the train had sliced in two as it ran over her. It seems likely, therefore, that as Kalamagyi fell under the train, she thrust her right leg out under the wheels, and it was cut off before other parts of her body were injured. If she did not lose consciousness immediately, she probably had done so by the time the train ran over her trunk.

Ma Khin Mar Htoo was born with her right leg absent from a few inches below the knee. Two rudimentary toes protruded from the stump of the leg (Figure 25). She had some minor defects of her hands, but they were trivial compared with the major defect of her leg. This condition, hemimelia in medical terms, is a rare malformation.

When Ma Khin Mar Htoo could speak, she expressed many memories of the life and death of Kalamagyi. Because the two families had been moderately well acquainted before the case developed, I do not believe Ma Khin Mar Htoo was able to say anything of which members of her family had no knowledge whatever. She developed a strong attachment to members of Kalamagyi's family and enjoyed visiting them.

This is one of the few cases in which we have been helpful to the subject in a concrete way. When we first met Ma Khin Mar Htoo, she was hobbling around on crutches, which had produced hard calluses on her hands. It was difficult for her to attend school. U Win Maung arranged for her to be fitted with a prosthesis, and when we last met her, in 1984, she was walking normally, able to climb stairs, and attending school successfully.

This chapter of the monograph includes four cases in which the subject remembered the previous life of a Japanese soldier killed during World War II. I presented summaries of three such cases in Chapter 4 and will now describe another.

Ma Win Tar was born in Pyawbwe, Upper Burma, on February 17, 1962. Her parents were U Aye Kyaw and his wife, Daw Khin Win. At her birth she was found to have severe defects of both hands. The middle and ring fingers of her right hand were present, but only loosely attached to the rest of the hand, and they were webbed together. A doctor recommended that these dangling fingers be amputated, and this was done when Ma Win Tar was a few days old. Several of Ma Win Tar's other fingers were either missing or had constriction rings. There was a prominent ring around her left wrist, and close examination of this showed that it consisted of three separate depressions that might have corresponded to grooves made by a rope wound three times around the arm (Figure 26). Daw Khin Win said that there had been a similar ropelike mark above Ma Win Tar's right wrist, but this had since faded. She also said that when Ma Win Tar had been younger, it was possible to discern in this area a pattern within the birthmarks that corresponded to the strands of the rope. (Figure 1 shows such rope patterns in a man who developed ropelike marks on his skin after vividly remembering having been tied with a rope some years earlier.)

Ma Win Tar started to speak when she was about 1½ years old. When she was about 3, she began to refer to a previous life. She said that she had been a Japanese soldier, captured by some Burmese villagers, tied to a tree, and burned alive. She gave no name for herself in the previous life, and her account of it remains unverified.

It is, however, plausible. As the Japanese Army retreated before the British advance in the spring of 1945, Burmese villagers would sometimes capture straggling Japanese soldiers. The stragglers were treated variously, according to the experiences the local villagers had had with the occupying Japanese Army. If the villagers believed the Japanese had badly mistreated them, they might take revenge on captured Japanese soldiers; and a Burmese associate who had been living in Pyawbwe at the time told me that some stragglers from the Japanese Army had been burned alive.

Ma Win Tar showed some behavior that was unusual in her family, but appropriate for the previous life that she claimed to remember. She liked to dress like a boy and to wear shirts and trousers. (Burmese boys, outside a large city like Rangoon, ordinarily wear shorts until they begin to wear the ankle-length garment known as a longyi.) She also liked to keep her hair short like a boy's. Eventually, her family forbade her to wear boys' clothes and insisted that she dress like a girl.

Ma Win Tar also showed several behaviors that I call "Japanese" traits. She complained that the Burmese food was too spicy and refused to eat spicy foods when she was young. She liked sweet foods and pork. She was relatively insensitive to pain and more hardworking than the average Burmese child. She had a streak of cruelty rare in Burmese children, and she sometimes slapped the faces of her playmates when they annoyed her. (This was a habit that the Japanese soldiers often showed when Burmese villagers irritated them; Burmese people rarely slap faces.) Ma Win Tar also resisted learning the forms of worship practiced by Burmese Buddhists. She refused to perform the customary gesture of obeisance when meeting Buddhist monks, despite the urgings of her parents. When Ma Win Tar was young, she would sit on the ground with her knees forward and her buttocks resting on her heels, as Japanese people do and Burmese people do not (except sometimes, briefly, when worshipping).

The behavior I have described certainly made Ma Win Tar stand out from her siblings and other playmates. It would not necessarily have alienated her from them if she had been less fervent, almost defiant, in insisting that she was Japanese. She would sometimes say: "I am Japanese. What do you think of me?" When members of the Japanese War Graves Commission came to Pyawbwe, Ma Win Tar told her playmates: "They are our nationals."

These attitudes led to quarrels in the home, and Ma Win Tar formed the idea that other members of the family were aligned against her because, as she put it, she was "a foreigner." I do not think her suspicions were warranted; on the contrary, I believe members of her family treated her kindly, even though Ma Win Tar's behavior must have tried their patience sorely.

When I last met Ma Win Tar in 1984, she had adjusted fully to life in Burma and said that she did not wish to "return" to Japan. She then had no imaged memories of the previous life, but she retained some masculine traits.

Augustine Nwachi, an Igbo, was born in Ndeaboh, Nigeria, in December 1977. His parents were Godfrey and Rebecca Nwachi. Augustine was born with a severe birth defect of his left foot. The outer third of the foot was absent. There were a few nubbins attached to the end of the stump that suggested attempts at toes (*).

Mainly on the basis of his birth defect, Augustine was identified as the reincarnation of his paternal grandfather, Dominic. The latter had died from an infection of his left great toe and second toe, which had become gangrenous, and must have culminated in an overwhelming infection that killed him within a few days of his becoming ill. From what I learned about the parts of Dominic's toes that had been affected, the diseased area of his foot was smaller than the substantial part of the foot that was absent when Augustine was born.

The Igbos attach importance to the judgment of an oracle concerning the identification of a reincarnated person, and in Augustine's case an oracle confirmed Godfrey's opinion that Augustine was the reincarnation of his (Augustine's) grandfather.

Augustine never spoke of any imaged memories of his grandfather's life or death. He thus belongs to an important group of subjects who undermine the idea, sometimes expressed by skeptics, that parents who identify a child as being a deceased person reincarnated will stimulate the child to express pseudomemories of that person's life.

Augustine's case has the additional importance of suggesting the value of the concept of a field in understanding how some of the birth defects I am describing occur: The area of his foot affected in the birth defect was considerably larger than the area involved in the infection of Dominic's foot.

By this time readers will have become used to the idea for the birthmarks figuring in these cases that there is not always an antecedent wound to which they correspond. Sometimes the body of the concerned previous personality had blood left on it or medicine spilled on it, or it was marked with lipstick or charcoal; in such cases the skin surface was not even scratched, let alone deeply wounded. In one case the generating factor for a birth defect was not even a mark on the previous personality's body; instead, it seems to have been a thought in his mind.

The case in question is that of Bruce Peck, a Haida, who was born in Massett, British Columbia, Canada, on November 20, 1949. His parents were Kenneth and Rose Peck. Bruce's paternal grandfather, Richard, was a renowned fisherman. In his day there was much less machinery for handling the fishing lines and nets than is available now. For the most part, lines had to be let out or hauled in by hand. It was heavy work, and Richard found the life of a fisherman unendurably severe. Three informants told me independently that they had heard Richard say that if he were reborn he wished not to have a forearm, so that he could not become a fisherman, and he would then be able to work at some less arduous job on land. As he said this, he gestured with his left hand straightened out making a motion like an axe coming down on his right arm and chopping it off below the elbow.

Richard Peck drowned accidentally on April 12, 1949. Bruce's mother was already pregnant at that time, and Bruce was born 7 months after his grandfather's death. The lower half of his right forearm was absent (*). At the end of the stump of his arm some nubbins of beginning fingers were present, and a surgeon later removed these.

Bruce had no imaged memories of his grandfather's life or death. No one had a dream before his birth. He did have a severe phobia of water. He worked entirely at clerical positions on the shore.

Readers of the numerous accounts of murders figuring in the cases I have already described will surely have noted that, if we interpret these cases as instances of reincarnation, it is the reborn victim who has birth defects, not the murderer. This can offend our sense of justice. Why, we may ask, should someone who is murdered also suffer from birth defects in another life? Outrage at such a thought led the mother of the murdered Yasupala in the case of Sampath Priyasantha (Chapter 3) to reject the idea that the horribly malformed Sampath Priyasantha could be the reincarnation of her son. In answer to this objection we can say that we do not know what happens to most murderers, if they should reincarnate. In a very few cases that have come to my attention, however, a subject who remembered having been a malefactor has had an apparently related birth defect.

One of the rare cases of this type I have investigated is that of H. A. Wijeratne. He was born in the village of Uggalkaltota, Ceylon (now Sri Lanka), on January 17, 1947. His parents were Tileratne Hami and his wife, Huratal Hami. At his birth Wijeratne was quickly noted to have marked birth defects of his right chest and arm. The major muscle of his right upper chest was absent, his right arm was much reduced in size compared with the left one, and the fingers of his right hand were extremely short; some of them were webbed together (Figure 27). (His condition, first described in the medical literature of the 1840s, is known as Poland syndrome.)

After Wijeratne began to speak, his mother heard him talking to himself. She became interested in what he was saying and, listening to him, was surprised to hear him say that he had been born with a defective arm because he had murdered his wife in a previous life.

When Huratal Hami told her husband what Wijeratne had been saying, she did not find him surprised. On the contrary, he had already surmised that Wijeratne was his late younger brother, Ratran Hami, reborn.

Ratran Hami had, in fact, told Tileratne Hami before he died that he would return as his son. In 1927 Ratran Hami had been engaged to a girl, Podi Menike, with whom he had gone through the preliminary ceremony for a marriage according to the prevailing custom of the time in what was then Ceylon. Podi Menike, however, had then changed her mind and refused to complete the marriage and return with Ratran Hami to his village. He had then walked back to his village, borrowed money to pay off some debts, sharpened a large knife (kris), returned to Podi Menike's village, and killed her.

Ratran Hami was beaten up by other persons present and arrested. After a trial he was sentenced to death and duly hanged in July 1928. (The interval between Ratran Hami's death and Wijeratne's birth is thus more than 18 years, much longer than that in most cases.)

Tileratne Hami was not married at the time of his brother's death. Readers puzzled over why Huratal Hami was surprised when she overheard Wijeratne's first utterances to himself should remember that Tileratne Hami, during his courtship and later, was unlikely to have told his wife about the criminal conduct and execution of his younger brother. All that had happened many years before and was best forgotten, he must have thought. I believe Huratal's statement that she knew nothing about the murder of Podi Menike until Wijeratne spoke about it.

At his trial, Ratran Hami had pleaded "not guilty" and offered an explanation of acting in self-defense along classical lines. He said that he had been set upon by persons present at Podi Menike's house and in the ensuing melée he had stabbed her. As we have seen, Wijeratne did not believe this. He freely acknowledged his guilt in killing Podi Menike and believed he was paying a penalty for the murder by being reborn with a malformed right arm. Yet he was not forgiving of Podi Menike. He was 14 years old when I first met him, and I asked him what he would do if he found himself in circumstances similar to those of Ratran Hami. He said that he would kill a girl who behaved as Podi Menike had done toward Ratran Hami.

This was not, however, his final view of the matter. I continued to meet Wijeratne from time to time when I was in Sri Lanka. In 1969 he wrote to me and said that on considering further how a man should respond to misbehaving wives he had decided that it was better to divorce than murder them.

Wijeratne's early life was far from uncomplicated. He seems not to have been self-conscious about his birth defect. He was, however, aware that girls might be reluctant to marry a man reputed to have killed his wife, even if he had done this only in a previous life. In 1969 he became mentally ill and was diagnosed as having schizophrenia. He completely recovered from this illness, persisted in his studies, and eventually qualified as a schoolteacher. He also married, and when I last had news of him, in 1982, he was happy and in good health.

18

BIRTH DEFECTS OF THE
HEAD AND NECK

The monograph reports 12 cases whose subjects had birth defects of the head and neck. From these I have selected 4 cases to summarize here.

Semih Tutuşmuş was born in 1958 in the village of Şarkonak, Karaağaç, in the province of Hatay, Turkey. His parents were Ali and Karanfil Tutuşmuş. Two days before Semih's birth, Karanfil dreamed of a man called Selim Fesli, who had been shot at close range in the head and had died of his wounds a few days later. In the dream the man's face was covered with blood, and he said that he had been shot in the ear. He also said that he was going to stay with the dreamer. Karanfil had never met Selim Fesli, although she had heard vaguely about his death. Her husband, Ali, had known him well.

Semih was born with a severe birth defect of the right ear. The external ear was represented only by a linear stump (Figure 28). In addition, the right side of his face was underdeveloped; in medical terms, it showed hemifacial hypoplasia.

Selim Fesli was a farmer who possessed a modest tract of land near a village called Hatun Köy, which is about 2 kilometers from Şarkonak. At the end of a day's work he was tired and lay down to rest and perhaps sleep before he left his fields and went home. In the twilight a neighbor, İsa Dirbekli, who was out hunting, mistook Selim Fesli for a rabbit and fired his shotgun at close range. He then heard Selim Fesli groaning, but instead of helping him fled from the scene, apparently fearful of being attacked by Selim Fesli's sons. Eventually, villagers found the wounded man and took him to a hospital in İskenderun, where he died 6 days later. We obtained a copy of the postmortem report on Selim Fesli, and it described penetrating shotgun wounds of the right parietal and frontal areas of the skull. The shots had entered the brain, and death was attributed to the wounds of the brain.

Semih began to talk about the life of Selim Fesli when he was about 1½ years old. His first words on the subject were the names of İsa Dirbekli, the man who had shot Selim Fesli. Thereafter, he stated more details about how, as Selim Fesli (whose name he gave as his own), he had been shot in the ear. He remembered also, and stated, the names of Selim Fesli's wife and all six of their children. Among 15 statements that Semih made about the previous life, 11 were correct, 2 incorrect, and 2 unverified. Because Selim Fesli was well known to Semih's father, I am not asserting that Semih made any statements including information that he might not have acquired normally. This does not mean that he did acquire his information normally, only that we cannot be sure that he did not. In addition to his statements, Semih was also credited with having recognized members of Selim Fesli's family and other persons known to him.

Semih had a strong desire to visit Selim Fesli's family. When he was still less than 4 years old, he found his way alone to Hatun Köy and introduced himself to members of Selim Fesli's family there. Later, he continued visiting the Fesli family and showed a strong attachment to its members. In Hatun Köy, Semih appears to have conducted himself like the father of the family and to have been, at least to some extent, accepted as such by its members. When one of Selim Fesli's sons was married, Semih was not invited to the wedding—possibly from oversight. Semih became annoyed at this neglect and would not speak to the Fesli family for two months. When another of Selim Fesli's sons became engaged and then married, Semih raised some money that he contributed to the bridegroom.

Semih showed an attitude of extreme hostility toward İsa Dirbekli. İsa Dirbekli had been arrested and tried for the killing of Selim Fesli. He pleaded that the shooting was entirely accidental. He was sentenced to 2 years in prison. After his release, he returned to Hatun Köy, where he set up as a vendor of rakı. He worked beyond his own village and sometimes came into Şarkonak. Semih believed that İsa Dirbekli had deliberately shot Selim Fesli. When he would see İsa Dirbekli, he would throw stones at him. He intended minimally to break İsa Dirbekli's bottles of rakı, and perhaps to break his head and kill him. He openly told us that he intended to kill İsa Dirbekli. İsa Dirbekli took these threats seriously—even though Semih was then only a young boy—and stayed away from the area of Şarkonak where Semih lived.

Reşat Bayer, who worked with me in the investigation of the case, tried to persuade Semih to adopt a more forgiving stance. He pointed out that if Semih had been Selim Fesli in a previous life he was now alive again as Semih. This argument availed little with Semih. He recognized its basic wisdom, but said that nevertheless whenever he saw İsa Dirbekli he could not prevent himself from wanting to throw stones at him and beat him up.

Semih continued in this vengeful attitude until the time came for him, at the age of 18, to perform his 2 years of compulsory military service. In the army a plastic surgeon constructed for Semih a remarkably normal-appearing external right ear. In addition, this improvement coincided with a change in hair styles, and Semih began to wear his hair long. Thus he no longer had any visible defect. This, in turn, seems to have enabled him finally to abandon the idea of revenging himself on İsa Dirbekli.

Süleyman Çapar was born in 1966 in the village of Madenli, south of İskenderun, in the province of Hatay, Turkey. His parents were Habib and Hekime Çapar.

Hekime dreamed during her pregnancy with Süleyman that a man on horseback approached her. She asked him why he was coming to her. He replied: "I was killed with a blow from a shovel. I want to stay with you and not with anyone else." Hekime later said that she did not recognize the man in the dream, and she seems to have given it little attention at the time.

When Süleyman was born, the back (occipital) part of his skull was depressed, and it had a prominent birthmark (*).

Soon after Süleyman began to speak, he pointed away from his house and said that he wanted to go to "the stream." Thereafter, beginning with fragmentary allusions, he gradually told details about a previous life. He described how he had been a miller and had been killed during a quarrel with a customer about which one of several waiting customers should have their grain milled first. One day, his mother, responding to Süleyman's wish to go to "the stream," let him show the way to a village called Ekber, where there was a stream and a mill. (Ekber is about 2 kilometers southeast of Madenli, although the distance is longer by road.) A little later, Süleyman's father took him on a second visit to Ekber, and on this occasion he met the mother of the man whose life Süleyman seemed to be remembering.

Süleyman had given the name Mehmet as the one he had had in the previous life. With the details of the profession of miller at the village of Ekber, it became clear that Süleyman was speaking about the life of a miller called Mehmet Bekler. Mehmet Bekler was born in Ekber in about 1940. When he grew up and had completed his obligatory military service, he returned to Ekber and operated the flour mill that his family owned. It was a water mill located on a stream outside the village. It is certain—from the medical records that I examined—that Mehmet Bekler died after being struck on the back of the head with a flour shovel. What had happened before that is unclear, because in the trial of Mehmet Bayrakdar (the man accused of killing Mehmet Bekler) all the resources of legal defense were used to obtain his acquittal. It seems, however, that when Mehmet Bayrakdar arrived at the mill other customers were already waiting to have their grain milled. He insisted impatiently that his need for flour was greater, and he even went so far as to pour some of his grain into the funnel of the running mill. Seeing this, Mehmet Bekler stopped the mill. The quarrel then became physical. Who struck the first blow is immaterial. Mehmet Bayrakdar hit Mehmet Bekler on the head with a flour shovel. Mehmet Bekler was transported to the Government Hospital in İskenderun, and he died there on November 28, 1965. The postmortem report included the following statement: "...a portion of the skull of the approximate size of the palm of the hand was fractured and depressed about a centimeter." Death was attributed to "subarachnoid hemorrhage due to trauma to the head."

Although the distance between the villages of the two families concerned in this case is short, the families had no personal acquaintance. Süleyman's family used a mill in Madenli and had no need to go to Ekber. Süleyman's father said that he knew Mehmet Bekler by sight only, and Hekime did not know him at all. Mehmet Bekler's mother said that she had not known the Çapars before the case developed.

I tabulated 18 statements that Süleyman made about the previous life. Of these 14 were correct, 1 incorrect, 1 doubtful, and 2 unverified. Habib Çapar said that when Süleyman had been younger he had stated additional names of the previous family members that, by the time we interviewed him, Habib could no longer remember.

Süleyman liked to visit Ekber, and he exchanged numerous visits with Mehmet Bekler's family. For their part, the Bekler family seem with one exception to have accepted Süleyman's claim to be Mehmet reborn. The exception was Katibeh Bekler, Mehmet Bekler's mother. She had acknowledged the accuracy of Süleyman's statements and had indeed been our principal independent verifier for many of them. Although she did not deny that Süleyman might be Mehmet reborn, she said she was not convinced that he was. I was unable to learn more about the reasons for her opinion; but because Süleyman had shown a somewhat possessive attitude toward the Bekler property, she may have imagined that he would claim some of it and tried to ward off this possibility by dissociating herself from his claim to be her son reborn.

Süleyman expressed considerable anger toward Mehmet Bayrakdar and said that when he was older he would kill him. Once, when he saw Mehmet Bayrakdar in Madenli, he pointed to him and said angrily: "He killed me." On at least one occasion, he asked his father to give him a gun so that he could shoot Mehmet Bayrakdar.

Maung Myo Min Thein was born in the village of Wundwin, Upper Burma, on September 14, 1967. His parents were U Aung Maw and Daw Thoung Nyunt.

When Maung Myo Min Thein was born, he was found to have a prominent birthmark—an area of hairlessness—at the back of his head (*). The observation by his parents of this birthmark did not lead immediately to his being identified with the man whose life he later remembered.

The first indication that Maung Myo Min Thein was remembering a previous life came when he was only 8 months old and his parents took him to the nearby Thein-gottara Monastery, where they had planned to pass the entire day in religious observances. At the monastery, Maung Myo Min Thein became frightened and began to cry. His parents could not pacify him, and they returned home.

When Maung Myo Min Thein became older, he tried to express memories of a previous life before he could do so properly with words. He would point in the direction of the Thein-gottara Monastery and show by gestures that he had been hit on the head. He was then about 3 years old.

By the age of 4 or 5 Maung Myo Min Thein had sufficient vocabulary so that he could narrate details of the previous life about which, up to this time, he had only given suggestions. He said that he had been the Ven. U Warthawa of Thein-gottara Monastery and that he had been hit on the back of the head with a heavy door bolt. When Maung Myo Min Thein said this, his parents examined his head more closely and found a depression on the back of his head that they apparently had not noticed earlier (*).

Maung Myo Min Thein made a few other statements about the previous life. He mentioned that his assailant had been a stranger to the monastery and also that he was mad. He also recalled that (not long before his death) he had asked one of the monks at the monastery not to make a journey to Mandalay that he had been planning; but the monk disregarded his wishes and went anyway.

Maung Myo Min Thein's statements were all correct for the circumstances of the death of the Ven. U Warthawa, who had been the much respected abbot of the Thein-gottara Monastery. A monk who was a stranger had come to the monastery one day, and the Ven. U Warthawa offered him its hospitality. No one appears to have noticed that the monk was mentally deranged. The Ven. U Warthawa knelt down in the temple of the monastery to worship before the image of the Buddha. With no motive that anyone later understood, the stranger monk struck the Ven. U Warthawa on the back of the head with a heavy bolt of the kind used for closing large doors. Stunned, the Ven. U Warthawa called for help, but before anyone could come to him, the stranger monk had taken a gong mallet and struck the Ven. U Warthawa on the back of the head with it. A general scuffle then ensued in which, in addition to the Ven. U Warthawa, another monk of the monastery was killed, and so was the stranger monk who had attacked the Ven. U Warthawa.

Maung Myo Min Thein showed a large number of behaviors—I tabulated eight in all—that were unusual in his family, but appropriate for the life and death of the Ven. U Warthawa. He continued to show the fear of the Thein-gottara Monastery that he had first manifested when only about 8 months old. Some of this fear persisted at least up to the age of 8 years. He showed a strong aversion to unfamiliar monks, a fear that seems to have been part of his memory of having been killed by a strange monk. He showed a distinct coolness toward the Ven. U Zawtika, the monk who had disregarded the Ven. U Warthawa's wishes and left for Mandalay shortly before the Ven. U Warthawa's murder. Maung Myo Min Thein thought that if the Ven. U Zawtika had remained at the monastery, the Ven. U Warthawa would not have been murdered.

As a young child, Maung Myo Min Thein liked to sit with his legs crossed in the habitual posture of Buddhist monks. (The posture is not exclusive to them.) More significantly, he chose a better and higher place on which to sit and would not sit on the empty rice-bags spread on the floor, where the rest of the family sat. This behavior indicated his identification with the role of a monk. Laymen who visit Buddhist monks (in countries of Theravadin Buddhism) are always expected to sit on the floor or on some chair or stool that is lower than the place where the monk is seated.

The Ven. U Warthawa had been keenly interested in music and theatrical productions, which he had both written and produced. Maung Myo Min Thein played with theatrical dolls and set up a miniature toy stage. He presented plays with dolls and other toys.

The Ven. U Warthawa died on April 1, 1949. The interval between his death and Maung Myo Min Thein's birth was therefore more than 18 years, one of the longest among the cases that I have investigated.

Maung Htoo was born in April 1978 in the village of Sipin Tabetkar, near Pyawbwe, in Upper Burma. His parents were U Kyaw Maung and Daw Win Kyi. Maung Htoo was born with a cleft lip (*) and cleft palate (*). When he was a young baby, he cried continuously unless one of his parents held him in their lap. When he was about 1½ years old, they used their savings to have Maung Htoo's cleft lip repaired, and when this was done he stopped crying.

When Maung Htoo was about 2 years old, he began speaking and soon made a number of statements that led his parents to suspect that he was remembering the life of Daw Win Kyi's uncle, U Paw Kywe.

U Paw Kywe had also lived in Sipin Tabetkar. He had worked first as an assistant to a truck driver and then as a pony-cart driver until he became ill with leprosy and no longer able to work. He had been married and had three children. The leprosy particularly affected his nose and adjoining parts of his mouth. His voice became nasal, which indicated that his palate had become eroded. His appearance became repellent, and his wife, Daw Aye Kyi, deserted him. She moved to Pyawbwe, taking their children with her. Thereafter U Paw Kywe lived alone. From fear of becoming infected, the villagers increasingly shunned him. In this extremity his last remaining friends were Daw Win Kyi and U Kyaw Maung. They would bring him food and water, which they left in a place from which he could reach it. This assistance was the more touching because U Paw Kywe had strongly disapproved of his niece's marriage to U Kyaw Maung. When U Paw Kywe saw that U Kyaw Maung, far from bearing a grudge against him, was fetching water for him, he apologized to U Kyaw Maung and asked forgiveness for the harsh language that he had used.

U Paw Kywe had a good friend, Ko Mya Win, whom he liked to visit. Not wishing to spread his disease, however, he did not enter Ko Mya Win's house. Instead, he would sit on a stone outside the house and converse with Ko Mya Win from there.

One day in 1976 Daw Win Kyi and U Kyaw Maung went to visit U Paw Kywe and not seeing him or hearing any sound from within the house, they entered it and found that he had died. With some other villagers they managed to give U Paw Kywe's body a proper burial.

Maung Htoo's birth defects corresponded—at least in anatomical region—to the part of U Paw Kywe's face that had been particularly destroyed by leprosy. As I mentioned, his cleft lip was repaired when he was an infant; and in 1987, when I last had word about him, his parents were planning to take him to Taunggyi for the closure of his cleft palate.

Like many subjects of these cases Maung Htoo at first lacked the vocabulary to express adequately what he wanted to say about the previous life. (His cleft palate also made it difficult to understand him.) He pointed toward the east and told his mother that he came from that direction. He said the words "Aye Kyi" and pointed toward the house of U Paw Kywe, whose wife, Daw Aye Kyi, had returned from Pyawbwe and was then living in the house. He held up three fingers for his mother and said: "I got three," meaning that he had three children.

Later, Maung Htoo spoke about some other details in the life and death of U Paw Kywe. He remembered that U Paw Kywe had been buried in the plastic sheet on which he had slept. (The villagers had done this in order to avoid touching the infected body.) He recalled an accident with U Paw Kywe's pony-cart that occurred 10 years before his death. And he remembered that bees had stung U Paw Kywe when he was working at the Sipin pagoda.

Maung Htoo showed much attachment to U Paw Kywe's old friend, Ko Mya Win, and liked to visit him. He recognized the stone where U Paw Kywe had sat when he visited Ko Mya Win.

When U Paw Kywe's younger brother, U Chit Maung, came to Sipin Tabetkar, Maung Htoo went up to him and addressed him in a manner that was familiar and appropriate for an older brother speaking to a younger one, but totally disrespectful in a young boy of 7 speaking to an older man who was a stranger. U Chit Maung took no offence at Maung Htoo's behavior. He said that U Paw Kywe had addressed him in exactly the same manner; and he became convinced that Maung Htoo was his older brother reborn.

U Paw Kywe's oldest son also accepted Maung Htoo's claim to be U Paw Kywe reborn; but his wife and daughter seem not to have done so. I was advised that Daw Aye Kyi would not cooperate in an interview, and I did not try to meet her. I conjecture that she may have been ashamed at having left her husband when he became seriously ill, but I obtained no direct evidence of this.

19

BIRTH DEFECTS INVOLVING TWO OR MORE REGIONS OF THE BODY

Ten cases do not fit appropriately into the chapters on birth defects of the extremities and of the head and neck; the subjects of these cases had defects and sometimes birthmarks involving two or more regions of the body. I will present brief accounts of four of these cases.

Ma Htwe Win was born in the village of Kyar-Kan, in Upper Burma, in May 1973. Her parents were U Shein and Ma Ohn Tin. Before Ma Ohn Tin became pregnant with Ma Htwe Win, she dreamed that a man who appeared to be walking on his knees, or perhaps on amputated stumps of legs, was following her; she tried to avoid him, but he continued to approach her. She did not recognize the man.

When Ma Htwe Win was born, her parents immediately observed that she had severe birth defects as well as prominent birthmarks. The birthmarks were on her lower left chest in the region of the heart (*) and on her head. The fifth finger of her left hand was absent (*). She had constriction rings around the lower parts of her legs above the ankles and another, particularly deep, constriction ring around the middle of her left thigh (Figure 29).

Ma Htwe Win's parents had no explanation for her birth defects and birth-marks until she began to speak. She then supplied one. She said that she had been a man called Nga Than and that three men had attacked him. He had tried to fight back, but when he made a thrust with his sword it got stuck in the wall, and he was left defenseless. They stabbed him in the left breast, cut his fingers, and hit him on the head. His assailants evidently thought they had killed him. In fact, Nga Than seems to have remained conscious for a time, so that Ma Htwe Win later remembered hearing the murderers drinking while they discussed how best to dis-pose of the body. They finally decided to compress it into as small a space as pos-sible by tying the legs back on the thighs, which would appreciably shorten the body and make it easier to put in a gunny sack and drop in a nearby dried-up well. Ma Htwe Win's statements were correct, so far as they could be verified, for the life and death of a man called U Nga Than.

U Nga Than's wife, Ma Hla Ohn, who had been a party to his murder, let it be known that he had left her and gone to the south. With the body safely disposed of, there was no reason for the police to be interested in a man who was absent because he had simply left his wife.

Ma Hla Ohn then married one of the murderers, but she was not happy with him. One day she and her new husband were drinking and quarreling, and in the course of their exchanges they mentioned the murder of U Nga Than and what they had done with his body. A neighbor overheard this conversation and went to the police, who then took a different view of U Nga Than's absence from the area. They went to the abandoned well and pulled out the body of U Nga Than, which was still tied up with the ropes that had been used to make it more compact.

The well where U Nga Than's body had been placed was near the road link-ing Kyar-Kan and the main road between the towns of Meiktila and Thazi. It hap-pened that Ma Ohn Tin was returning from the main road to her village when she noticed a small crowd. Its members had gathered around the police, who were just at that moment bringing up U Nga Than's body and untying it. Ma Ohn Tin glanced at the body and ropes and went on her way. She was then about 2½ months pregnant with Ma Htwe Win; and the dream that I mentioned earlier occurred during the night following her view of the exhumation of U Nga Than's body.

In addition to her statements, Ma Htwe Win spontaneously recognized one of U Nga Than's murderers, who was still in the area, and she showed consider-able fear of him. She also recognized U Nga Than's son and asked her parents for some money that she could give him.

Ma Htwe Win showed some masculine traits, such as a wish to wear boys' clothes. Her mother would not allow her to do this. She also expressed a determi-nation to revenge herself on the murderers of U Nga Than. She was distressed by her birth defects. One day, stretching out her legs to show their defects, she said to her grandfather: "Grandpa. Look at what they did to me. How cruel they were."

If Ma Htwe Win's legs were folded back behind her thighs, the constriction rings on her lower legs would be at the same level as the deep constriction ring on her left thigh. We have no verification of exactly how U Nga Than was tied up, but these constriction rings are certainly concordant with what Ma Htwe Win said about how U Nga Than's body was tied up before being put in the well.

The tying of the legs in the fashion Ma Htwe Win described may also explain the dream that Ma Ohn Tin had of a man walking on knees or stumps. This figure would correspond with the mental image of his body that the deceased U Nga Than might have had after his body was put in the well.

Thiang San Kla was born in the village of Ban Rasai, near Surin, in Surin Province, Thailand, on October 9, 1924. His parents were Charon and Puen San Kla.

Charon and Puen had both dreamed before Thiang's birth that Puen's deceased brother Phoh had appeared to them and said that he wished to be reborn as their child. At Thiang's birth or soon afterward, he was found to have six birth defects and birthmarks, which I shall describe later. These, together with his parents' dreams, made them think that Thiang was Phoh reborn. Phoh had died about a year before Thiang's birth.

Phoh San Kla had been a notorious cattle thief, and one day when he went to a village where a number of his enemies had gathered, they attacked and killed him. He was hit on the back of the head with a heavy knife of the kind that Thai villagers use for opening coconuts or chopping wood. The blow probably killed Phoh instantly. Members of Phoh's family, including both of Thiang's parents, went to the village where Phoh had been killed and viewed his body, which was buried in that village 3 days after his death. This occurred in October 1923.

Some time before his death, Phoh had injured his right foot in an accident. His right great toe became infected and never healed before he died. It apparently suppurated, because his sister Ping later told me that Phoh's right great toe smelled badly.

Thiang's two major birth defects corresponded respectively to the fatal wound on Phoh's head and the chronic infection of his right great toe. On the back of the left side of his head, Thiang had an extensive lesion that in medical terms was a verrucous epidermal nevus (Figure 30). When I examined it in 1969, it was slightly raised above the surrounding skin, hairless, heavily pigmented, and much wrinkled. It was irregular in shape and measured about 5-6 centimeters long and 1-1.5 centimeters wide. The defect of Thiang's right great toe consisted of a partially detached portion of the nail of that toe, and this nail or the tissue beneath it was darkly pigmented (Figure 31). Thiang's other birthmarks were of lesser importance in the investigation of the case, because they had faded by the time we studied it. They were said to have been marks on the backs of his hands and the insteps of his feet that corresponded to tattoos on Phoh.

Thiang was less than 4 years old when he began to speak about the life of Phoh. We know that he was not older, because his father died when Thiang was about 4, and he had become convinced before he died that Thiang was Phoh reborn. (Part of his conviction, however, would have derived from the dreams that he and his wife had and from Thiang's birth defects.)

A policeman who had investigated both Phoh's cattle thieving and his murder learned that Thiang was claiming to be Phoh reborn and went to see him. He later told us that Thiang at once recognized him and called him by name. Thiang also correctly stated to him the names of the persons who had killed Phoh. Thiang himself told us that Phoh's wife, Pai, also visited him and tried to test his knowledge of Phoh. She brought with her a number of articles that had belonged to Phoh as well as some that had not. Thiang said that he easily sorted out the articles that had belonged to Phoh and that he also narrated to Pai incidents of their married life. Pai had died by the time of our investigation, so we could not independently verify Thiang's account of their meeting. We could, however, interview Phoh's daughter, Pah. She said that Thiang had spontaneously recognized her and called her "daughter." He convinced her that he was her father reborn by his detailed memories of Phoh's life and death. Thiang was about 7 years old at this time. Another of our informants said that Thiang had laid claim to some land adjoining an army camp, on the grounds that it had belonged to Phoh. He correctly stated the circumstances in which Phoh had acquired the land. I need hardly say that an adjudicating court rejected his claim.

As a young child Thiang said his name was Phoh, and he would sometimes become angry if he was called Thiang instead of Phoh. He sometimes called his father "brother" and called his paternal aunt "sister," instead of "aunt."

Thiang had no phobia of knives, and he seems also to have had no fear of the village where Phoh had been killed. He did, however, show a markedly vengeful attitude toward the people who had killed Phoh. He told me that even in middle adulthood he sometimes had fantasies of going to the village where Phoh had been killed and there killing any of Phoh's murderers who might still be living.

In honesty of character, however, Thiang differed from Phoh. He made a good soldier during a period of service in the Royal Thai Army, and afterward he returned to his village, where he eventually became its respected headman. His memories of the life of Phoh with reflections on his misdeeds and death led him to resolve to be a better person.

Ariya Noikerd was born in Bangkok, Thailand, on November 7, 1968. Her parents were Hong and Nitaya Noikerd. Before Ariya's birth both her mother and her mother's older sister, La-Mom, dreamed that Apirak, a son of the family who had been killed 3 months earlier, was going to return to the family. Nitaya dreamed that Apirak asked permission to come back, but in La-Mom's dream he only said that he would be reborn in the family. Ariya was born about a year after Apirak's death.

When Ariya was born, she was quickly found to have a widespread port-wine stain birthmark on the left side of her face and head (*). In addition, she had an unusual cleft or deep crease in the skin of her lower back, near the midline and just above her right buttock (*). Apirak had had an exactly similar cleft at the same site.

To understand the port-wine stain birthmark on Ariya's face and head, we must go back to Apirak's death. He was a boy of just 13 when he went with his family on a visit to the town of Pakchong, 180 kilometers northeast of Bangkok. While there he (and some other persons) were struck by a truck. Apirak was killed almost instantly. Apirak's grandfather was injured, but other members of the family escaped. Because Apirak was killed in Pakchong, his body had to be transported from there to Bangkok. There was some mismanagement in this, but in due course, 7 days after his death, his body was cremated in Bangkok. In the meantime, it had not been washed, and blood remained on the face and head where it had been right after the accident. I did not learn, and Apirak's parents probably did not know, from what injury or injuries Apirak had died. I do not know that he was injured in the head, but think this probable. Both of Apirak's parents and his maternal aunt (La-Mom) said that the birthmarks on Ariya's face and head were at exactly the places where blood had been on Apirak's face when his body was cremated.

Apirak had been a distinctly girlish boy. Although he did not refuse to wear boys' clothes, he liked to wear girls' clothes, and when he did so he would apply rouge, lipstick, and eye makeup to his face. He wore girls' clothes so often that his mother remembered him more as thus dressed instead of wearing boys' trousers. He seemed to her also to have a feminine gait. He often played girls' games, and most of his friends were girls. He had said at least once that he would like to be reborn as a girl.

Apirak seemed somewhat depressed and several times expressed a wish to die. When reproached for having such thoughts, he said that he wanted to know what happened after death.

Apirak's only other relevant trait was a fondness for dancing to drums.

I think I reached this case sooner after it developed than any other that I have investigated. Ariya's parents were convinced on the basis of the announcing dreams and Ariya's birthmarks and birth defect that she was Apirak reborn before she had said a word. An account of the case appeared in a Bangkok newspaper in December 1968, and I went to visit Ariya and her family in March 1969.

At that time Ariya was still less than 5 months old. In 1971 I continued the study of the case, and by this time Ariya had made a few statements about the life of Apirak. After that, I lost touch with the family for a time, but found them again in 1980.

When Ariya spoke about the previous life, she did so only in response to questions, and at least one of these was a leading one. She did, however, communicate that the birthmarks on her head came from a "wound by the car." And she identified a photograph of Apirak as one of "Ut," which was Apirak's nickname. Her maternal aunt mixed some of Apirak's toys and clothes that the family had kept with other similar items and asked Ariya to select those that had belonged to Apirak. She said that Ariya did this successfully.

Ariya seems not to have had a phobia of trucks when young, but in 1980 I learned that she then did have a phobia of them. She showed markedly masculine behavior and preferred wearing boys' clothes instead of girls' clothes. In 1980 her preference for wearing boys' clothes was continuing. At the age of about 2½ Ariya spontaneously began to dance when she heard drums. Her family noticed this and thought it suggestive of Apirak's interest in dancing to drums; but I did not learn that Ariya showed this interest on later occasions.

Like most port-wine stains, Ariya's did not fade as she became older. Both the birthmark on her face (*) and the cleft near her buttocks (*) were just as prominent in 1980, when she was 11½, as they had been when I first saw her as a baby only a few months old.

This is the third case in which informants have attributed birthmarks to blood left on the previous personality's body when it was cremated: The other two were those of Sunita Singh and Narong Yensiri. A somewhat similar case is that of Ma Chit Chit Than, in which a birthmark corresponded to spilled medicine.

Sukh Lal Sharma was born in 1908. The case is therefore very old. Moreover, I never met Sukh Lal, who died in 1943. I did, however, meet his older brother, Samokhi Lal, and another villager of Bisalpura, Madhya Pradesh, India, where Sukh Lal had been born and lived. Moreover, a careful Indian investigator, R.B.S. Sunderlal, studied the case when Sukh Lal was about 10 or 12 years old and in 1924 published a report of it in a French scientific journal. In order to get to know Sukh Lal well, he had kept him in his house for a week. He had also studied police reports concerning the murder of a man called Kashi Ram, whose life Sukh Lal remembered when he was a child.

Kashi Ram had been a tax collector, and he became involved in a case for tax evasion against a man called Chhotey Lal, who came from a nearby village, Nonenhta. Chhotey Lal tried to win Kashi Ram over to his side, but Kashi Ram proved incorruptible. Chhotey Lal shot Kashi Ram in the chest, and then, while he was still alive, he mutilated Kashi Ram's hand. The murder occurred near the above-mentioned villages, which are in the extreme northern part of what was then the princely state of Gwalior (now part of the state of Madhya Pradesh). Chhotey Lal fled from the scene of the murder, managed to escape into British territory, and was never prosecuted. Kashi Ram was murdered not more than a year before Sukh Lal's birth.

I obtained from Samokhi Lal what I believe is a satisfactory description of Sukh Lal's birth defects. His right chest had a deep concavity (*). His right hand had only a stump of the thumb and no other fingers except the little finger, which was essentially normal; part of the palm of the hand was absent (*). (Although I have indicated that the monograph includes figures of Sukh Lal's birth defects, these are not photographs but artist's sketches made from the descriptions of the defects.) Sunderlal stated that Sukh Lal's birth defects corresponded to "the description of the dead body in the police file."

When he was a young child, Sukh Lal said that his name had been Kashi Ram and that he had been killed by Chhotey Lal. When asked about the birth defect of his right hand, he said that "kakka" had cut it. ("Kakka" was a nickname for Chhotey Lal.) Sukh Lal remembered details of the last minutes of Kashi Ram's life. He said that after Chhotey Lal shot him in the chest, he cut off the fingers of his right hand except for the little finger. He mutilated the hand because it had been writing out tax bills; but he spared the little finger because it had not been involved in holding the pen that wrote the bills.

Chhotey Lal, who had later returned to the area, learned of Sukh Lal's statements and went over to see him. He was standing in a crowd of people when Sukh Lal recognized him and called out that Chhotey Lal was his enemy and murderer.

The birth defect of Sukh Lal's right hand is an extremely rare one and occurs in about 1 in 150,000 births.

20

EXPERIMENTAL
BIRTH DEFECTS

This chapter could be considered a sequel to Chapter 10, in which I described cases of experimental birthmarks. The difference is that in experimental birth defects the bodies of deceased persons are not just marked, but mutilated in some way, and later-born babies with birth defects are said to be these babies reborn; informants say the birth defects correspond to the mutilations on the deceased baby.

The practice of mutilating certain dead babies occurs across the entire extent of sub-Saharan West Africa, from Nigeria in the east to Senegal in the west. It derives from the belief in the cultures of this region that children who die have a major responsibility for their deaths. (This attitude differs markedly from the one prevailing in the West, according to which, when a child dies, blame becomes attached to the child's parents or doctors, or, if they seem faultless, to God or chance.)

In West Africa two or more successive deaths of infants in the same family lead the parents to believe that the same soul is returning to them, only to die, be reborn, and die again. These are then called "repeater children," and to stop such a useless and vexatious cycle of rebirth and death, the parents sometimes mutilate a recently deceased child. They believe that this inculcates the lesson that the misbehaving soul of the child should either go away and never come back or, if it returns to the family, stop dying in childhood and grow up. Sometimes parents suspect children who are physically frail or significantly ill of being repeater children. In such cases they may carry out, or have someone else carry out, a sort of preemptive mutilation of the child to prevent it from dying.

Details of the belief in repeater children and of the mutilations practiced vary among the different ethnic groups of West Africa, but what I have described should suffice for the understanding of the three cases that I will now summarize. They all occurred among the Igbo of Nigeria.

Among the Igbo a child thought to be a repeater child is called an *ogbanje*. In the region around Awgu, in Anambra State, children suspected of being an ogbanje sometimes have the last part of the left little finger amputated as a means of preventing them from dying. When Dr. Stuart Edelstein and I were in Awgu in 1981, we asked the principal of a school to show us some children who had had parts of their fingers amputated for this reason. Within a few days he found and showed us 13 such children.

All but one of the children had definite scars on the stumps of their short-ened left little fingers, but one had no scar. He was Onuchukwu Nwobodo, and we studied his case further.

Onuchukwu's father said that he had been born (in about 1968) with both of his fifth toes absent (*) and the end part (distal phalanx) of his left little finger also absent (*). Onuchukwu never spoke about a previous life. His father was our sole informant for the case, and we reviewed with him conjectures about a previ-ous life that Onuchukwu might have had.

It had been suggested that Onuchukwu might have been the reincarnation of his paternal grandfather, but this proposal included no explanation of Onuchukwu's birth defects. A more plausible explanation was that he had had a previous life as an ogbanje and had been mutilated after dying. If so, this life could not have been as a child in his own family, because before Onuchukwu's birth they had had no child die. Several cousins had been considered ogbanjes, and Onuchukwu might have had a previous life as one of them. None, however, was identified as Onuchukwu's previous personality.

Cordelia Ekouroume was born in Umuokue, Imo State, Nigeria, in 1958. Her parents were Ekouroume Uchenda and his wife, Irodirionyerku. Cordelia was born with some of the most severe birth defects of the hands, legs, and feet that I have ever seen (*). Most of her fingers and toes were short and had no nails. Some were webbed together. Her lower legs had constriction rings. Her father, who was our sole informant for the case, explained them in the following way.

Ekouroume Uchenda had a sister, Wankwo, who believed herself to be mis-treated by a man and asked her brother for help. He told us that he was a skilled sorcerer and that he obligingly killed the man who had offended his sister, not with ordinary physical violence, but with sorcery.

Some time afterward, Wankwo died. Ekouroume Uchenda believed that one of his next children was Wankwo reborn, and he welcomed her back into the family. Then, however, this baby died in infancy. Ekouroume Uchenda became enraged at the ingratitude of this child—the reincarnated Wankwo, he believed—in dying so young. He considered that he had been badly repaid by his sister after all the trouble he had taken to remove by sorcery a man who had mistreated her. In his anger he chopped off the fingers and toes of the dead baby. Then, symbolically to prevent it from ever walking again, he tied a rope around its legs. As he was carrying out these mutilations, he spoke to the soul of the dead baby (and, he believed, that of his ungrateful sister) and told it never to return. To enforce this proscription, he put some of the baby's chopped off fingers and toes in a little bag, which he hung up in his house.

Following these events Ekouroume Uchenda—who, like many Igbo men, was a polygamist—married another junior wife, Irodirionyerku. She knew little or nothing about the history of her husband's sister and the baby he thought was his sister reborn. One day she was cleaning the house and noticed the little bag of the baby's remnants that Ekouroume Uchenda had hung up. Thinking it of no importance she threw it away. She happened to mention the matter to her husband, who was horrified at what she had done, because he believed she had broken the spell by which he had sought to prevent his sister from ever again being reborn in their family. He was afraid that his wife's next baby would be seriously malformed. He proved correct, because this next baby was Cordelia.

Ekouroume Uchenda assured us that Cordelia's birth defects corresponded to the mutilations he had made on the dead baby that he believed had been the reincarnation of his sister. We do not need to believe that he precisely remembered each finger and toe that he had cut off the baby; but I have no reason to doubt that he was correct in general when he told us that Cordelia's birth defects corresponded to the mutilations that he had made on the dead baby.

Cordelia, I was told, never spoke about a previous life. We were not permitted to interview her, partly, it would seem, because she was understandably sensitive about her birth defects. Yet she stood cooperatively while I examined and photographed her.

Florence Onumegbu was born in Isieke-Ibeku, Imo State, Nigeria, in about 1942. Her parents were Dick Onubugo and his wife, Hannah.

When Florence was born, she was quickly found to have severe birth defects of both her feet and both her hands. The last thirds of both feet, including the toes, were absent (*). The fingers of both hands (except for the thumbs) were markedly shortened, and most had no nails (*).

Florence's father had died before I investigated this case, and her mother, Hannah Dick (whom I tried to interview), was a reluctant witness. Most of the Igbo are formally Christians, and, although most of them that I came to know did not believe that Christianity conflicts with their traditional religion, some did; and Hannah Dick was one who did. She preferred not to discuss events that had occurred "when she had been a pagan."

My principal informant for the case was, therefore, Florence's husband, Timothy Onumegbu. He was necessarily a secondhand witness for the main events of the case; he assured me, however, that he had had considerable hesitation about marrying a woman with birth defects as serious as those of Florence. He therefore took much trouble to interrogate the persons directly involved in the case before he made up his mind to marry Florence. (I did not learn why he believed that he should make such an inquiry, but he may have been thinking that Florence's defects might be inherited by any children they would have.)

One of Florence's uncles and his wife had had several children who died in infancy. The uncle, angered by this succession of infant deaths, had mutilated the body of the last dead baby. Florence was born not in the family of the uncle, but in that of his brother.

Timothy Onumegbu told us that he had learned that Florence's birth defects corresponded to the mutilations her uncle had made on his dead baby.

Florence had no imaged memories of a previous life. Her own five children were normal.

21

INTERNAL DISEASES RELATED TO PREVIOUS LIVES

Compared with the abundance of cases whose subjects have birthmarks and visible birth defects, I have found few subjects with internal diseases that corresponded to a similar disease in a person whose life the subject claimed to remember. I can identify several possible explanations for this, but there may well be others of which I am unaware.

First, some feature of the skin and the more exposed parts of the body, such as the extremities, head, and neck, may make them more susceptible to the impact of wounds (and other marks) than are the internal organs. Second, the birth defects certainly, and most of the birthmarks that I have described in these cases, are obvious at a baby's birth and easily noticed then or soon afterward. In contrast, most diseases of the internal organs develop slowly and only manifest in later childhood or adulthood. By this time most subjects of these cases have forgotten the previous life, and the life of the previous personality lies even farther back in time. Informants may fail to make a connection between a later-developing illness in the subject and a similar one from which the previous personality suffered. Third, in the countries where I have found most of these cases, medical facilities are still not well developed; moreover, informants of these countries are less knowledgeable about the details of illnesses that they or their family members may have than is the average layperson in more developed countries. Consequently, when I have asked for the cause of someone's death, I have often been able to learn no more than that he or she died of "some fever" or "old age." Finally, the comparative meagerness of our data about internal diseases may derive from my own early neglect of this aspect of the cases when I first began to give attention to birthmarks and birth defects.

Even so, I have notes of some relevant observations of internal diseases, and when I came to tabulate these, I found that in 25 cases the subject had shown symptoms that were similar to ones from which the concerned previous personality had suffered. In some of these cases the subject showed the relevant symptoms in childhood for a few months or years only, and then, as we sometimes say, he or she "outgrew" them. For example, a subject of Burma, Maung Tin Aung Mo, who remembered the life of a man who had died from a pulmonary disease, probably tuberculosis, coughed a great deal when he was an infant and was suspected of having tuberculosis; but this condition cleared by the time he was 3 years old. I will summarize here two of the cases for which we have the most evidence.

Maung Aung Myint was born in Moulmein-gyun, Burma, on October 22, 1967. His parents were U Thoung Shwe and Daw Khin Shwe. Before Maung Aung Myint's birth, Daw Khin Shwe had two dreams that suggested to her the rebirth as her child of a cousin, Maung Mya Maung, who had been killed when Daw Khin Shwe was pregnant.

When Maung Aung Myint was born, he was quickly observed to have a prominent birthmark under his right nipple (*). He also had a large nevus on his lower back (*). The birthmark near his right nipple corresponded to a fatal chest wound that had killed Maung Mya Maung about 3 months before Maung Aung Myint's birth. The nevus corresponded to a nevus that Maung Mya Maung had had at the same site. In later childhood, Maung Aung Myint developed "red urine," which I believe resulted from blood in his urine (hematuria); Maung Mya Maung had suffered from urinary disease, and I will discuss these abnormalities later.

Maung Mya Maung was born in 1936. When he was a young child, he remembered a previous life and satisfied informants that he had real memories of it. Maung Mya Maung became a hotheaded and pugnacious young man. One day, when he was intoxicated, he and an acquaintance, Maung Kyaw Lay, began quarreling and continued angrily until Maung Kyaw Lay challenged Maung Mya Maung to a fight with swords. This quickly embroiled their friends, who were also armed. Maung Mya Maung and a single friend then advanced to meet their adversaries. They found that they were badly outnumbered by the opposing gang. Maung Mya Maung decided to take the offensive and charged at his opponents. One of them was armed with a kind of long spike, and he drove this into Maung Mya Maung's chest. Maung Mya Maung was taken to the Rangoon General Hospital, where he died a few hours later. I was unable to examine the record of his admission to the hospital, but I obtained satisfactory testimony from firsthand witnesses concerning the correspondence in location between the wound on Maung Mya Maung's chest and the birthmark on Maung Aung Myint's chest; I must mention here, however, that the birthmark was just below the nipple and could be considered an auxiliary nipple.

When Maung Aung Myint was less than 2 years old, he began to speak about the previous life of Maung Mya Maung. Because the two families concerned were related and near neighbors, I do not believe that he can have said anything outside the normal knowledge that his parents (and he) would have had of the life and death of Maung Mya Maung. Maung Aung Myint did not remember the anterior life that Maung Mya Maung had remembered when he had been young.

Maung Aung Myint showed a strong identification with Maung Mya Maung and addressed persons Maung Mya Maung had known by the familiar names that would have been customary for him but that were disrespectful when spoken to elders by a young boy. He also had strong vengeful thoughts toward Maung Kyaw Lay, whose nephew had driven the fatal spike into Maung Mya Maung's chest.

Maung Mya Maung had suffered from "urinary disease" that was not further specified. Maung Aung Myint had frequent attacks of "red urine," which was almost certainly due to blood in the urine (hematuria). I was able to examine a record of a treatment he had had in an outpatient clinic for "urinary obstruction." This suggests urinary stones (calculi) as a cause for the "red urine."

Selma Kılıç was born in 1959 in Adana, Turkey. Her parents were Yusuf and Latife Kılıç. When Selma was born, she was quickly observed to have a large red birthmark in the skin of the left side of her lower back (*). When she first began to walk, her mother noticed that she tended to keep her hands on her back and over the area of the birthmark. Neither the birthmark itself nor Selma's tendency to put her hands on it made any sense to Latife Kılıç until Selma was found, at the age of about 7, to have kidney disease.

Selma was about 2½ years old when she first began to refer to a previous life. Her opening statement occurred when she went out onto the street before her family's house and said that she wanted to find "my mother." When Latife said that she was Selma's mother, Selma replied: "No. You are not my mother." She insisted on being allowed to go to "my mother" and eventually had to be forcibly carried back inside the house.

Selma persisted in her demands to be allowed to go to "my mother," and eventually Yusuf Kılıç suggested to Latife that she let Selma go where she wanted and follow her. Latife did this, and Selma led the way through the streets until she came to a place near a public water fountain, where she said: "There! I have found my mother." Latife, dismayed and perhaps frightened, picked Selma up and took her home. On the following day, Selma's grandmother, with Latife's consent, took her back to the public water fountain. From there Selma found her way to a house where she went up to a woman whom she embraced, saying: "Here is my mother."

Selma's grandmother and the woman Selma addressed as "my mother" exchanged some information. The woman had had a daughter who had died of kidney disease, and this seemed relevant to Selma's birthmark in a way that impressed the woman, who began to cry.

This woman was Emine Zaman, and her daughter, Zehra, had died at the age of about 17 or 18, of kidney disease, in 1958.

It turned out that the two families concerned in the case had had some acquaintance before it developed. Latife knew Zehra Zaman's sister, Kadriye, and when she next met Kadriye she mentioned Selma's identification of Kadriye's mother as "my mother." Kadriye decided to meet Selma and went to see her. Selma recognized her immediately and then described to Kadriye's satisfaction numerous details about the last months, illness, and death of Zehra Zaman. Kadriye later remembered 12 statements that Selma made to her about the life of Zehra, and they were all correct but one, which was doubtful.

I did not obtain a medical record of Zehra's illness, but she was described as having widespread swelling of her skin, and her water intake had been restricted, which indicate that she had edema, of which kidney failure is an important cause. One informant said a doctor in Istanbul diagnosed Zehra as having nephritis, and another said that a doctor in Adana had said she had "a kidney disease."

For Selma's illness I was able to obtain firsthand evidence. A doctor had first told Latife that Selma had kidney disease when she was about 6 or 7 years old; but I do not know on what symptoms he based this statement. Over the next few years Selma continued to be somewhat sickly and complained of pain in the region of her kidneys. In 1969 she was admitted to the Government Hospital in Adana, and we were able to study her medical records of that admission. Her discharge diagnoses were "gastroenteritis" and "acute glomerulonephritis." The laboratory examination of her urine showed that it contained protein and many red blood cells. Selma continued to have symptoms of kidney disease up to the time of our last information about her, in 1975, when she was 16 years old.

Selma talked often about the previous life when she was young and continued doing so beyond the age when most subjects stop referring to a previous life. Visits with Zehra's family did not sustain Selma's memories, because the visits did not continue after perhaps two occasions. I conjecture that her illness might have kept her memories more in her consciousness than would have occurred if she had been in good health. Among statements that she made to us in 1970, when she was about 11 years old, some were correct, but others were not and appear to have been elaborations and distortions. In the monograph, I have listed and discussed these inaccurate statements.

22

Abnormalities of Pigmentation That May Derive from Previous Lives

In this chapter I present a group of cases the subjects of which showed pigmentation that was unusual in their family and that corresponded or, in unsolved cases, may have corresponded to similar pigmentation in the person whose life an affected subject remembered. Suggesting that a person's entire pigmentation may derive from a previous life seemed to me, and still seems, more complicated and controversial than pointing out correspondences between wounds and birthmarks or birth defects. Readers should know that I investigated these cases with great skepticism and for a time even considered omitting them from the monograph.

In preparation for reporting the cases of this chapter, I reviewed the medical literature about hair that was said to turn white suddenly or, as the saying goes, "overnight," as a result of some extreme fright. I thought that if hair really can turn white overnight from some sudden emotional disturbance, this would be evidence that a mental cause could alter pigmentation, presumably through a disruption in the metabolism of melanin, which is the principal pigment of the skin. Most dermatologists believe that hair does not turn white overnight; the idea that it does, they believe, arises from the falling out—admittedly often from a psychological shock—of ordinarily pigmented hair. Previously existing white hair is left behind, and its new prominence produces an illusion that the subject's hair has "turned" white suddenly. This explanation may well apply to some cases. There remain other cases, however, to which it could not apply. I refer to instances that were closely observed by competent witnesses who reported no loss of hair in the person affected at the time the person's hair was observed to turn white suddenly. Furthermore, I found two well-documented reports of cases in which subjects had suddenly lost the pigment of part of the skin of their faces (*). I also found one case reported by a physician in which maternal impressions offer the only plausible explanation for the occurrence of albinism in some, but not all, of a mother's children.

When I examined notes that I had made of cases that I had investigated, I found that no fewer than 14 of the subjects had been reported to have had pigmentation that differed from that of other members of their family but corresponded to that of the person whose life a subject remembered.

U Kalar was a subject who showed a comparative increase in pigmentation. I have not met him, but one of my assistants sent me a report of his case, and another one sent me a photograph showing U Kalar with his brother; and the photograph clearly shows that they had markedly different pigmentations.

U Kalar was born in the village of Soo-dut-gyi near Tawngdwingyi in Upper Burma in (about) 1942. His name means "dark" in Burmese, and his parents so named him because of his complexion and because they believed, as I shall explain, that he had been an Indian in a previous life.

When U Kalar was about 3 years old, in the spring or perhaps summer of 1945, he saw some British soldiers who had returned to Burma after defeating the Japanese Army toward the end of World War II. The British soldiers stimulated memories of a previous life in U Kalar, and he then narrated the following details.

He said that he had been a soldier in an Indian regiment of the British Army during its retreat before the Japanese. (This would have been early in 1942. The British had then been pushed back as far as Tawngdwingyi. Eventually, they retreated all the way to India.) The Indian soldier whose life U Kalar was remembering and a companion went off from their company in search of alcohol. Some Burmese villagers offered them drinks and invited them to come to their village, Soo-dut-gyi. Then the villagers got them helplessly drunk and attacked them. (The Burmese villagers presumably wanted the soldiers' weapons.) The Indian soldiers tried to escape, but were caught and killed. The villagers left their bodies where they had killed them.

Soon after, U Kalar's father, U Maung Sein, happened to pass in his bullock-cart, and he noticed the bodies. He thought they should not be left there and transported them to a place away from the village. U Maung Sein told his wife about the dead Indian soldiers. Later, his wife dreamed that one of the Indian soldiers came into the house and said he had come to stay with them. Not long afterward she became pregnant with U Kalar.

No one could verify U Kalar's statements about how the Indian soldier had been killed, but his father said he was correct in describing how he (the father) had found and removed the soldiers' bodies from where they had been left by their murderers. In order to help readers understand this case, I will remind them that the Burmese are an Indo-Chinese people, and their complexions are nearly always fairer than those of Indians.

U Kalar showed a darker pigmentation compared with other members of his family. I come next to cases in which changes in the opposite direction occurred that amounted, in some of them, to albinism.

Archana Shastri was born in Srinagar, Jammu and Kashmir, India, on November 7, 1964. Her parents were Netra Pal and Bhagwati Devi Shastri. Archana was appreciably fairer than other members of her family; her irides, in particular, were said to have been blue when she was born, although they later became a light yellow-brown (*).

When Archana was still a young child, she expressed a longing to go to "her home." She gradually brought out details of a previous life in which, she said, she had been a wife and mother of several children. The whole family had gone for a vacation to a resort hotel that had been destroyed, along with its residents, in a sudden flooding of the river near which it stood.

Archana's statements reminded her family of a great flood (in Kashmir) in which many people had lost their lives some years earlier. A Moslem family, slightly known to Archana's, had been among the victims drowned in the flood. Archana met members of this family and satisfied them that she had memories of the life of one of them, Tahira Khanam.

As a young child Archana showed Moslem habits, such as saying the Moslem prayer (namaz) five times a day.

Tahira Khanam, whose life Archana remembered, had been fair and had had blue eyes.

B. B. Saxena was born in Bareilly, Uttar Pradesh, India, (probably) in 1918. His parents were Ram Charan Lal and his wife, Sudama Kunwar. At his birth B. B. Saxena was noted to be extremely fair in complexion. His hair was almost white, although his irides were brown (Figure 32). He had two prominent birthmarks, one on his neck, which was roundish and looked somewhat like a bullet wound of entry (Figure 33), and another, a hairless scarlike area, at the top of his head (*).

B. B. Saxena began to speak about a previous life when he was between 3 and 4 years old. He said that his name was Arthur and that he had been a "white" soldier who died in "the German war" (World War I). He said that he had two brothers and a mother; his father had died long ago. He himself was a Captain in the Army and died in a battle, during which he was on horseback. (B. B. Saxena pointed to the birthmark on his neck as he mentioned his death in the previous life.) He had been married to an English wife; they lived in a house with a kitchen and employed a cook.

All this seemed strange to B. B. Saxena's parents. His father was a scrivener and law clerk who could not speak English and had little to do with the few English people settled at that time in Bareilly. B. B. Saxena's statements, however, surprised his family less than his behavior did. He played at being a soldier and strutted up and down giving military orders. He also played at games totally unknown to his Indian family, such as leapfrog and hopscotch. He did not like wearing Indian clothes, such as the dhoti, and wanted to wear shorts instead. For food he asked for bread and butter instead of the Indian *chapatti*. Although his family were vegetarians, he asked for meat. He complained about the cooking of vegetables in fat or butter and wanted his cooked in water. He objected to the chilies and spices so liberally used in Indian cooking. He did not wish to use his right hand in taking food to his mouth, as most Indians did and do, but called for a knife, fork, and spoon.

B. B. Saxena's parents suppressed him from speaking about the previous life, not because they disbelieved him, but because they superstitiously thought that children who remember previous lives die young. Fortunately, the case came to the attention of K. K. N. Sahay, a lawyer of Bareilly whose own son, Jagdish Chandra, had remembered a previous life. Sahay included a brief report of B. B. Saxena's case in a pamphlet in which he reported six other cases, including that of his son. He published this in about 1927. Many years later, I was able to meet not only B. B. Saxena, but also his older brother and older sister, both of whom remembered his statements and unusual behavior as a child.

As B. B. Saxena grew up, he forgot the imaged memories of the previous life, and he gradually became what I may call "Indianized." He nevertheless preserved into middle adulthood some traits that might properly be described as "British." For example, he still preferred to eat with cutlery instead of with his hands, ate bread in preference to rice, and never ate chilies.

In connection with other cases, I have often considered whether the subject's parents, noticing a birthmark, have decided that the subject is the reincarnation of a particular person and then, perhaps unwittingly, have imposed that identification on the child. I acknowledged earlier that this explanation has some force with many cases, and it may indeed be the correct one for a few of them. In the case of B. B. Saxena, however, I find it absurd. In the 1920s when B. B. Saxena was at the peak of making his statements and showing his "British" behavior, Gandhi's "Quit India" movement was steadily gathering force. No Indian family would have gained any merit by claiming to have an English Army officer reborn among their children. Apart from this, Ram Charan Lal and his wife would have had scant experience with the British from which they could have learned how to coach a child to imitate English behavior, especially the games that B. B. Saxena played, which were completely unknown to his family.

In conclusion, I will mention that the British Army had a cantonment in Bareilly during the period with which we are concerned in this case. Some soldiers from that cantonment served in France and later in Mesopotamia (now Iraq). It is therefore possible that B. B. Saxena remembered the life of a British soldier who, after having been stationed in Bareilly, had fought and been killed in World War I.

Before I began to investigate the cases of children who claim to remember previous lives, I had studied published reports of some cases, which I found mostly in somewhat obscure books and newspapers. Among these reports two from Burma described blond children who, to judge by the reports, had given convincing evidence of having been Englishmen in a previous life. Although precise dates were not given for the second case, I could estimate that the subject had been born in Meiktila, Upper Burma, around 1904. I thought that in the late 1960s he might still be alive. I therefore asked a correspondent, the late Dr. R. L. Soni, if he would make inquiries about this subject in Meiktila, which is about 120 kilometers south of Mandalay, where Dr. Soni lived. Dr. Soni said he would enquire about the case that interested me, and he did this. He did not find that case, but his informants brought him to the much more recent one of Maung Zaw Win Aung.

Maung Zaw Win Aung was born in Meiktila, Upper Burma, on May 9, 1950. His parents were U Tin Aung and Daw Kyin Htwe. He was the first of the 12 children they eventually had.

Maung Zaw Win Aung had a moderately severe degree of albinism. His complexion was fair and his hair blond (Figure 34). His irides were light brown. He had nystagmus (rapid involuntary eye movements) and also suffered from sensitivity to light (photophobia). Both these symptoms are typically found in albinism. In addition, the form of his eyes was much closer to the usual form of the eyes of Caucasians than it was to the usual form of the eyes of the Burmese, most of whom have eyes of Mongolian form (Figure 35). (In eyes of Mongolian form the distance between the eyelids tends to be less, and the fold of the upper eyelid is less prominent than in eyes of Caucasian form.)

Almost as soon as he could speak, Maung Zaw Win Aung began to say that he had been an American aviator whose airplane had been shot down and had crashed near Meiktila. He said he had a companion in the airplane, but there was ambiguity—perhaps due to limitations of the Burmese language—as to whether he remembered being the pilot of the airplane. (Because he later played at being the pilot of an airplane, we could suppose that he was then remembering this role.) Maung Zaw Win Aung made a number of other statements about the previous life of which the most important was that his name was John Steven. He also mentioned how he and his fellow pilots drank alcohol, sometimes when they were on bombing missions.

Maung Zaw Win Aung could not describe the airplane that he had been in when it crashed. Nor was he able to state the military unit to which he belonged, the rank he had, or the kind of uniform he wore. He did remember that the airplane he flew was not based in Burma. From the information that he furnished, it was not possible to trace any person corresponding to his statements. These were, however, plausible. American fighter-bombers, stationed at a base near Calcutta, aided the British as they advanced into Burma against the Japanese early in 1945. The fighting for Meiktila was particularly severe, and the Japanese shot down some of the American bombers. Maung Zaw Win Aung's statements were therefore credible, but in most details they remain unverified.

As a young child Maung Zaw Win Aung showed several behaviors that were unusual in his family but could be considered "Western," by which I mean that they harmonized with Maung Zaw Win Aung's statements that he had been an American aviator.

He was in the first place nostalgic for America and said he would return there if he could. He extolled America as a much better place in which to live than Burma. He expressed anger at the Japanese. He wanted Western types of clothing, such as shoes, trousers, and a belt. He was fascinated with airplanes and for many years said that he would later become a fighter pilot. As I mentioned, he played at being a pilot. He resisted taking food to his mouth with his hands (which nearly all Burmese people do) and ate with a spoon until he was about 12 years old. He did not like the spicy food of the Burmese and asked for milk and biscuits. He seems to have had a strong desire for alcohol, but he never expressed this as a young child.

A prominent feature of Maung Zaw Win Aung's behavior when he was a young child was an alternation in his moods. At times he would speak boastfully about the bombing raids in which he had participated. Then he would swing to an attitude of repentance and say that he had sinned in killing so many persons. He seemed to want to approach Buddhist monks as if they could give him absolution for his war crimes, as he then saw his conduct at such times. (At that young age he did not understand that there is no doctrine of forgiveness in Buddhism, but he might have mistaken the monks for Western priests; both groups wear long robes.)

As Maung Zaw Win Aung grew into later childhood and youth, he still had some memories of a better life in America, but he was obliged to confront the life he had to live in Burma. Sometimes he tried to escape from unpleasant features of the "present life" by dwelling on the memories of the previous one. They, however, made him sad and sometimes even seemed to bring on a severe chest pain. At our first meeting in 1970, he summed up his feelings by saying: "I am dominated by my surroundings." Eventually, he resolved to become fully Burmese, and I think he succeeded. He entered medical school, subsequently qualified as a physician, and then married. His marriage was a happy one, and at the time of my last information about them, he and his wife had had a son—of normal Burmese pigmentation and features.

When Maung Zaw Win Aung was about 10 years old, his mother dreamed that a Western woman came to her and asked to be born into her family so that she could be near her brother. Daw Kyin Htwe was pregnant at the time of the dream, and she later gave birth to a blond girl who was given the name Dolly Aung. Dolly Aung was also an albino. She was quite blond, although her irides were a light brown. She was short-sighted and suffered from nystagmus. The external form of her eyes was Caucasian (*).

Dolly Aung never spoke about a previous life. She did, however, exhibit some of the "Western" traits, such as in preferences of food, manner of eating, and desired clothing, that her older brother had shown. She was also strongly attached to him, as he was to her.

Daw Kyin Htwe subsequently gave birth to two more blond boys, each birth being preceded by a dream of a blond man. These children had eyes closer to the Caucasian than the Mongolian form. The older one also had shown some indications of "Western" traits, but both these later-born children were still young when I had my last contact with the family.

All four of the family's blond babies weighed appreciably more at birth than any of the other children, who had normal Burmese pigmentation. (Western people are, on average, appreciably larger and heavier than Burmese people.)

I know that this case lends itself to quick dismissal, even to ridicule. It can easily be concluded that U Tin Aung and Daw Kyin Htwe each carried a gene for albinism—each being, as geneticists say, heterozygous. (They produced albino children from four out of twelve pregnancies, close enough to what we should expect from genetic factors alone.) The parents, deciding these blond children must have been Westerners in previous lives, then guided them toward such an identification. I do not think this a sufficient explanation of all the facts of which we should take account. I am unable to believe that Maung Zaw Win Aung's parents had any desire, even if they had the capacity, to impose Western identifications on their children. But is any other interpretation better?

If we interpret the case as one of reincarnation or—taking account of all the blonds in the family—of several instances of it, we can imagine an American aviator being killed in Burma and reborn in a Burmese family; his sister and then two brothers or friends follow him into the same family. This explanation would account for the Caucasian form of the subjects' eyes and for their large weights at birth. What are we to make, however, of the severe degree of albinism, complete with ocular symptoms, that the blond children showed? We cannot imagine anyone with Maung Zaw Win Aung's visual disabilities qualifying to become a wartime aviator. In short, if Maung Zaw Win Aung did have a previous life as an American aviator, he might have been fair, but he could not have been an albino. So if we adopt reincarnation as an explanation for the case, we must acknowledge that in the process of being reborn the aviator overdid—bungled, in effect—the influence he had on the pigmentation of the baby in whose body he was to reincarnate.

Interpreted as instances of reincarnation, the cases of Archana Shastri on the one hand and U Kalar on the other suggest that a mental influence from a discarnate personality can induce slight to moderate diminutions or augmentations of pigmentation in embryos and fetuses. They presumably would do this by interfering with the metabolism of melanin at some stage. The commonplace phenomenon of suntanning teaches us how sensitive the processes of skin pigmentation are. Perhaps—still speculating about reincarnation—we may suppose that in certain instances the mental influence we are conjecturing damages the metabolic processes and interferes so much with the metabolism of melanin that albinism results.

In the monograph I describe seven other cases of blonds in Burma who communicated that they had been Westerners in a previous life or whose parents, interpreting what the children said and how they behaved, decided that they had been Westerners. Although these additional cases have less detail than those of B. B. Saxena and Maung Zaw Win Aung, they do add important data of which we must take account. Unfortunately, they do not seem to carry us toward any entirely satisfying interpretation of these cases. I am far from content with our understanding of them.

23

PHYSIQUES, POSTURES, GESTURES, AND OTHER INVOLUNTARY MOVEMENTS RELATED TO PREVIOUS LIVES

In preceding chapters I have sometimes drawn attention to examples of the features with which I am concerned in this chapter. For example, I described the left-handedness of Ma Khin Sandi and Corliss Chotkin, Jr. with the suggestion that this trait in them might have derived from the previous lives that they remembered or were thought to have had. I also mentioned the unusual gaits of William George, Jr. and Ma Myint Myint Zaw; and I drew attention to Ma Win Tar's habit of kneeling with her buttocks on her heels, as Japanese people do, but the Burmese ordinarily do not.

Although I gave little attention to these features during the early phases of my investigations of the children who remember previous lives, I later obtained a substantial amount of relevant data from which I will extract a few illustrative cases for this chapter.

Ma Khin Ma Gyi and Ma Khin Ma Nge were twins born in the Shan States, Burma, on February 5, 1961. Their parents were U Ba Thaw and Daw Mya Tin.

Before their births their mother dreamed that her parents were going to be reborn as her children.

When the twins were able to speak, they referred to the previous lives of their grandparents. Ma Khin Ma Gyi, who remembered the life of the grandfather, spoke more than Ma Khin Ma Nge, who remembered the life of the grandmother. (The detailed report of their case is in Chapter 25 of the monograph.)

As a young child, Ma Khin Ma Gyi showed markedly masculine behavior and insisted for many years on wearing boys' clothes. More remarkable for the topics of this chapter were the differences in the physiques of the twins. From analysis of their blood groups I learned that the twins were fraternal or dizygotic, that is, developed from two ova; therefore, their genetic material was not the same, as it is in identical (monozygotic) twins. Nevertheless, I think the differences in their physiques noteworthy. It was most easily seen in their legs. Ma Khin Ma Nge had thin, gracile legs, whereas Ma Khin Ma Gyi's legs were thick and stocky (*).

Dulcina Karasek was born (probably) in 1919 in Dom Feliciano in the state of Rio Grande do Sul, Brazil. Her parents were Patricio and Georgeta de Albuquerque.

I never met Dulcina, who died in 1937 at the age of about 18. I first learned about her case during my first visit to Brazil in 1962. Even though the case was then already old, I found and interviewed some informants who seemed reliable. Subsequently, I continued gathering information about the case until I believed I had enough to justify a report of it.

In early childhood Dulcina had frail health, but was otherwise not physically remarkable. She was somewhat later than most subjects in speaking about a previous life and may not have referred to it until she was 5 years old or even older. When she did speak about it, however, she spoke often and abundantly. I shall pass over most of what she said, which is not pertinent to the features of sex change and physique in the case.

Dulcina said that she was called Zeca, and she stated details about the life of a cousin of her parents called José Martins Ribeiro, who was generally known as Zeca. He had been born in about 1872.

As a young man Zeca had engaged in political and revolutionary activities and experienced adventures that figured in Dulcina's memories. Later, he established himself in a business in the town of Dom Feliciano and married. Then he became ill and died, perhaps of syphilis, in 1897 at the age of 25. His wife was pregnant at the time of his death and later gave birth to their only child.

Dulcina strongly identified with Zeca. She would say: "Do not call me Dulcina. I am Zeca, a man, and married." She repeatedly denied that she was a woman and insisted that she was a man. Once she asked her mother: "Why did I change my sex? I was a man and now I am a girl." On another occasion, she looked at herself in a mirror and, turning to her mother, asked: "Why did my eyes change color?" (Zeca had had blue eyes, but Dulcina's were brown.)

Dulcina preferred to wear boys' clothes instead of girls' clothes. It was observed that when she mounted a horse, she did so as a man would instead of as a woman.

As she became older, Dulcina developed a masculine physique. One feature of this came to attention when she was about 9 years old and became ill. In the course of her medical examinations, her doctor had an X-ray made of her pelvis. This showed that she had a distinctly small pelvic outlet. The doctor told Dulcina's father that she would not be able to deliver a baby in the normal way and advised him to have Dulcina sterilized; but this was not done.

After puberty Dulcina grew a great deal of hair on her arms, legs, and upper lip, where she had a noticeable moustache. One informant said that she was "full of hair," and another (who had known her well at school) said that she was "very muscular and quite masculine." Three out of four informants thought that her breasts were underdeveloped; the fourth did not think so.

Despite her masculine physique and gender orientation toward masculinity, Dulcina matured sexually and became enamored of a young man whom she married. She then became pregnant. As the doctor had predicted 9 years earlier, she was unable to give birth to the baby through the vaginal canal. She agreed to a cesarean operation, but immediately after the operation both Dulcina and her baby died.

Jim Bailey was a Tlingit who was born in about 1851 in Alaska. He was identified as the reincarnation of a man who had drowned at Yakutat not long before Jim Bailey's birth. I did not learn how this identification came to be made, but a dream may have contributed to it. Even more, the unusual posture of Jim Bailey promoted the identification. The posture, informants said, corresponded to the position the body of the drowned man had been in when it was retrieved from the water.

The unusual posture derived from permanent flexion of the legs. Jim Bailey could not stand erect, but remained all his life in a crouched-down position (*). His unusual posture led to his sometimes being called "the bear boy of Sitka." (He spent most of his life in Sitka.) He was normally strong in the upper parts of his body, and if a man would crouch down to Jim Bailey's level, he could wrestle with him on equal terms.

I believe that the previous personality of this case developed—at the time he drowned—the condition known as cadaveric rigidity. This occurs especially when death comes suddenly, as it often does in drownings. The muscles become rigidly stiffened.

Until a few years ago I knew of no case parallel to that of Jim Bailey, and I was unsure that I was correct in attributing cadaveric rigidity to the previous personality in his case. In recent years, however, I have studied two other cases showing close similarities to that of Jim Bailey. One occurred in Sri Lanka, the other in northern India. The previous personalities in both these recent cases had drowned; and in both cases the subjects assumed postures—one only when asleep, the other when awake—that corresponded to the postures in which the bodies of the previous personalities had been when they were retrieved from the water in which they had drowned. I believe they also had cadaveric rigidity.

Gillian and Jennifer Pollock were identical (monozygotic) twins of England. They were born on October 4, 1958. When they were between the ages of 3 and 7, they made a few statements and recognitions suggesting memories of the lives of their own older sisters, who had been killed in an automobile accident about 17 months before the twins were born. The older sisters had not been twins. The older, Joanna, had been 11 and the younger, Jacqueline, had been 6 when they were killed. Gillian remembered the life of Joanna and Jennifer the life of Jacqueline. (The detailed report of their case is in Chapter 25 of the monograph.)

Joanna, at 11, had been attending school for about 5 years and had learned to hold a pen and pencil properly. Jacqueline, however, had been attending school for only about a year before she died. She had adopted a way of holding a pen or pencil upright, enclosed in her fist. Efforts by her parents and teacher to teach her to hold a pen or pencil properly had failed.

When Gillian and Jennifer first learned to write, at the age of about 4½, Gillian immediately grasped the pencil properly. In contrast, Jennifer held the pencil upright in her fist, just as Jacqueline had done (*). I followed the cases of the Pollock twins for many years. Even in her twenties, Jennifer still sometimes held a writing implement in her fist.

24

THE FACE AS A
TYPE OF BIRTHMARK
OR BIRTH DEFECT

It may seem unkind and even rude to include a discussion of faces among chapters about birth defects. I have become convinced, however, that in some cases unusual facial features of a subject correspond to similar features in the face of the person whose life the subject claimed to remember. Unfortunately, as with physiques, postures, and gestures, I gave little attention to facial resemblances during the early years of these investigations. What I am able to present on the subject now will have value mainly as a guide for future investigators who should make a systematic study of this and other features of the cases the importance of which I came to appreciate late.

These facial similarities may occur under three different circumstances. First, an unusual facial appearance may correspond to severe damage to the face or its nerves in a previous personality. An example in this category occurred in the case of Semih Tutuşmuş (Chapter 18). Semih had a severe birth defect of his right external ear; in addition, the whole right side of his face was underdeveloped (hemifacial hypoplasia), and that gave it an asymmetrical appearance. Second, the face of a subject who remembers the life of a person from a different racial group may resemble the usual face of that group more than the usual face of his or her native race. Third, a distinctive facial feature of the subject, such as a sharply pointed nose or unusually prominent ears, may correspond to a similar feature in a previous personality.

A satisfactory study of similarities in the facial appearances of subject and related previous personalities should include photographs of both faces of a pair to be compared. Unfortunately, I have not often been able to obtain photographs of the previous personalities, but the monograph includes several cases for which I do have such photographs (*).

Ma Hmwe Lone was born in Inbetgone, Upper Burma, on May 21, 1953. She had a congenital paralysis of the left seventh (facial) cranial nerve, which gave a droop to that side of her face and prevented her from fully closing her left eye (*). She also had an extensive hairless scarlike birthmark on the left side of her head above and behind her left ear (*). (The detailed report of her case is in Chapter 18 of the monograph.)

Ma Hmwe Lone remembered the life of a man called Ko Hmwe, who was generally known as a rough, tough sort of person. He quarreled with another man at whom he threw a bomb, which failed to kill his adversary. The latter, armed with a sword, then struck at Ko Hmwe and hit him a fatal blow behind the left ear, killing him almost instantly.

Ma Hmwe Lone's facial paralysis might correspond to injury to the left facial nerve of Ko Hmwe from the blow that killed him. The nerve might have been damaged where it passed through the base of the skull or after it emerged into the softer tissues behind the face.

Maung Mhat Tin was born in Nga-Zun, Upper Burma, on February 27, 1945. (The detailed report of his case is in Chapter 9 of the monograph.) He remembered the previous life of a farmer called Maung Aung Su, who was conscripted by the Japanese Army (occupying Burma during World War II) to participate in the removal of bags loaded with rice from one town to another. A group of bullock-carts was to move together at night. In order to prevent pilfering of the rice each bullock-cart carried a Japanese soldier, who monitored the driver. The soldier on Maung Aung Su's cart harassed him to such an extent that Maung Aung Su took his sword, killed the soldier, and tipped the dead body off the bullock-cart. All this was unobserved as the line of bullock-carts continued to move ahead in the dark. The next morning, however, the Japanese discovered that one of their soldiers was missing. They quickly identified who had killed the soldier and sentenced him to be executed by a firing squad.

The Japanese executed Maung Aung Su in public, intending thereby to deter any other farmer from interfering with their activities. Maung Mhat Tin remembered that, to prevent himself from showing any fear in public, Maung Aung Su had bitten his lower lip just before he was shot. Maung Mhat Tin had birthmarks of increased pigmentation that corresponded to the bullet wounds that killed Maung Aung Su (*). In addition, his lower lip was grossly enlarged to the point of being slightly malformed (*).

Maung Soe Tun was born in Magwe, Upper Burma, on August 28, 1965. At or soon after his birth, the opening (palpebral fissure) of his right eye was found to be markedly narrower than that of his left eye (*).

After Maung Soe Tun became able to speak, he began referring to a previous life as a woman called Daw Soe, who was a friend of his mother. Daw Soe had lived and died in the town of Myinmu. Toward the end of her life she developed cataracts and had an operation for this on one eye. Maung Soe Tun said that he remembered that the right eye was the one operated on. He said that his vision was poorer in that eye than in his left one. My other informants could not remember on which eye Daw Soe had been operated. If I may reason backward from the birth defect to the related illness—a move that I do not ordinarily approve—I would say that Daw Soe's right eye was the diseased one operated on.

In the category of facial correspondences to the nation or race of the previous life, I have already mentioned the Caucasian form of the eyes of some of the blond and albino subjects in Burma who said that they were American or British flyers in a previous life or whose parents so identified them.

Similar observations were made about some of the numerous Burmese subjects who claimed to remember the previous lives of Japanese soldiers. The informants, but more importantly my long-time interpreter and associate, U Win Maung, remarked from time to time that one of these subjects "looked like a Japanese." Most Burmese and all Japanese people have eyes of the Mongolian form. I do not think that I am a reliable judge of the differences between the face of an average Burmese person and that of an average Japanese one. I respect U Win Maung's opinion sufficiently, however, to recommend a systematic comparative study of such facial differences, with judges who would not know which subjects claimed to have been Japanese in a previous life and which had not.

Maung Nyunt was born in Magyibin, near Tatkon, Upper Burma, on December 4, 1940. Both his parents were Burmese. After he became able to speak, he described the previous life of an Indian pony-cart driver. He said that he had been a Hindu. He gave no name for the Indian whose life he remembered, and the case is unsolved. Maung Nyunt recalled that somehow the pony-cart that he remembered driving tipped back so that the driver fell backward out of the cart, landed on his head, and died instantly.

Maung Nyunt showed when young a number of behaviors that were unusual in his family, but that were typical of Hindu Indians. He was born with symmetrically placed small areas of increased pigmentation at the backs of the helices of both ears (*). These birthmarks corresponded, it is supposed, to holes pierced for earrings, which Hindu pony-cart drivers habitually wore. (He was one of the nine subjects with similar birthmarks on the ears to which I referred in Chapter 8.)

I include this brief report of Maung Nyunt's case in this chapter because his facial appearance was noticeably more Caucasian than Mongolian in form. As I mentioned earlier, the Burmese are an Indo-Chinese people, and most of them have eyes of Mongolian form; Indians, on the other hand, are Caucasians and have eyes of Caucasian form. Unfortunately, the photograph of Maung Nyunt's face that I took did not bring out a difference that seemed definite to me when I looked at him (*).

Ma San San Nyunt and Ma Nyunt Nyunt San were twin sisters who were born in 1964 in the small town of Yanaung, Upper Burma. (The detailed report of their case is in Chapter 25 of the monograph.) After they became able to speak, they made a number of correct statements about the lives of two deceased sisters (not twins) who had been cousins of their father. The sisters were Daw Aye Phyu (the older sister) and Daw Sapai; and they had died—elderly women then—at separate times some years before the twins were born. Ma San San Nyunt remembered the life of Daw Sapai and Ma Nyunt Nyunt San remembered that of Daw Aye Phyu. I was able to obtain and copy photographs of the deceased women (*), which readers of the monograph can compare with my photographs of the twins (*). Those who do this will, I am confident, see a distinct resemblance between the faces of Ma Nyunt Nyunt San and Daw Aye Phyu and one between those of Ma San San Nyunt and Daw Sapai. The most obvious describable feature is the palpebral fissures, which were narrower in Daw Aye Phyu and Ma Nyunt Nyunt San than they were in Daw Sapai and Ma San San Nyunt. There also seems to me a definite similarity in the lower forehead and root of the nose in the faces of Daw Sapai and Ma San San Nyunt. They both show a slight frown that is absent in Daw Aye Phyu and Ma Nyunt Nyunt San.

If future investigators follow my recommendation to make a systematic study of facial resemblances between subjects and previous personalities, they will have to decide at what age of the persons concerned the faces should be compared. Informants have sometimes told me that a subject resembled the person whose life he or she remembered when young, but did not do so when the subject became older. This suggests that the faces of young children—when they are at the peak of speaking about a previous life—should be compared, when this is feasible, with photographs of the previous personalities not far from the time when they died.

25

TWINS WITH MEMORIES OF PREVIOUS LIVES

Since Francis Galton in the late 19th century first proposed the value of twins to help distinguish the effects of "nature and nurture," many studies of twins have been conducted with the aim of identifying the different influences of what we now speak of as "genes" and the "environment." In such studies, differences in concordance for certain diseases between identical (one-egg or monozygotic) twins and fraternal (two-egg or dizygotic) twins have been particularly clarifying. Monozygotic twins have the same genetic material; dizygotic twins are no more alike genetically than ordinary siblings. Significant differences between the two kinds of twins therefore should show the extent of genetic influence in a feature under study. In fact, monozygotic twins may have substantially different uterine experiences, and some differences between them may derive from these. The studies of twins who claim to remember previous lives suggest that other differences between monozygotic twins, and between dizygotic ones also, may derive from previous lives.

In earlier chapters I have referred to three twin cases: those of Ma Khin Ma Gyi and Ma Khin Ma Nge (Chapter 23), Gillian and Jennifer Pollock (Chapter 23), and Ma San San Nyunt and Ma Nyunt Nyunt San (Chapter 24). Later in this chapter, I will present accounts of three other twin cases. I will also add further information about the Pollock twins. First, however, I will describe some results of the analyses of all the twin cases in our collection.

My associates and I have investigated a total of 40 twin cases in which one or both twins spoke about a previous life. To these I have added two additional cases of which earlier authors published reports. There are therefore 42 cases of twin pairs and 84 subjects and 84 previous personalities to be considered. Some of our cases have not been as fully investigated as I should like, but the series is large enough so that we can draw at least some tentative conclusions from it.

I need to emphasize, however, that more than half our twin cases occurred in Burma. The large number of twin cases from Burma may derive partly from the large number of cases of all kinds that we have studied in Burma. The proportion of twin cases among all cases in Burma is, however, much higher than the proportion of twin cases among all cases in India. The overall rate of twinning is not significantly higher in Burma (about 12.5 per thousand births) than it is in the United Kingdom (11 per thousand births). It is possible that being a twin in Burma somehow facilitates the emergence of memories of a previous life. Be that as it may, I need to warn readers that the large contribution to the series of cases in Burma limits the generalizability of the results of our analyses. Burmese cases in general—not just the twin cases there—differ in some important respects from cases in other cultures. In particular, the incidence (26%) of cases of the sex-change type in Burma is much higher than that of cases of this type in most other cultures.

We were able to determine the zygosity—whether the twins came from one egg or two eggs—in six pairs of twins by analysis of their blood groups and subgroups. Only two pairs were one-egg twins (monozygotic). The series undoubtedly contains other one-egg twins, but unfortunately we do not know with assurance which ones these are. Close similarity of facial features so that the twins of a pair are often confused, even by persons who know them well, is a good indication of monozygosity; but difference in facial appearance is not a reliable indicator of dizygosity. One study showed that as many as 18% of twins who looked different were nevertheless monozygotic. Later investigations have shown lower figures for such inaccuracies, but it is safe to assume that 5% of twins who look different are in fact one-egg twins. (Indika and Kakshappa Ishwara, whose cases I summarize later in this chapter, are examples of monozygotic twins who did not look alike.)

Among the 42 cases, 71% of the twin pairs were of the same sex and 29% of different sexes, proportions not appreciably different from an estimate that I derived from a large study of the zygosity of twins in the United Kingdom. Among the 84 subjects, 18 (21%) remembered a previous life as a person of the opposite sex or were identified as having had such a life.

The subjects varied widely in the extent to which they spoke about previous lives. In 10 cases both twins spoke to the same extent; in 12 cases one twin said much more than the other; in 13 cases one twin spoke, but the other said nothing; in 2 cases neither twin spoke, but informants identified them as having had previous lives on the basis of dreams, birthmarks, and behavior. (For 5 cases we had no information on this feature.)

Among the 13 cases in which only one twin spoke about a previous life, in 6 cases the twin who spoke placed the silent twin in his or her previous life, that is,

claimed to have known him or her in previous lives during which they were con-
temporaries. For example, one twin (of Burma) said that in a previous life he had
been an officer in the British Army and that his co-twin had been his servant in the
army. The co-twin never spoke about a previous life, but he showed subservient
behavior toward the twin who spoke that was harmonious with the different statuses the one who spoke said they had previously had.

In another case of this type, also in Burma, the twins' mother dreamed,
about 1 month before she became pregnant with them, that a relative, one Ko
Than Aung (who had died 3 months earlier), said that he was coming to live with
her and was bringing a companion with him. One of the later-born twins, Maung
Kyaw Myint Naing, subsequently spoke about memories of the life of Ko Than
Aung. He also told his family that in the discarnate realm, where he (as Ko Than
Aung) found himself after death in the previous life, he had seen a villager, U
Saing (also discarnate), and had called to him to come along with him (to be
reborn as his twin). U Saing had been an inhabitant of the same village, but not a
relative of the family; he had died some time before Ko Than Aung. Maung Kyaw
Myint Naing's co-twin never spoke about the life of U Saing.

In 36 (86%) of the 42 cases the previous personalities had been related or
acquainted (or one twin said they had been). The relationships were of different
kinds. Some had been spouses, others siblings, and others more distant relatives,
friends, or acquaintances.

There was also a high incidence of a relationship or acquaintance
between the previous personalities and the twins' parents. Among the 84 previous personalities, 26 were related to the parents and another 26 were acquainted with them, so that there was some personal connection between the previous
personalities and the twins' parents in 62% of the cases. Another 15 previous
personalities were strangers to the twins' parents, and 17 may or may not have
been strangers.

There was a high incidence (56%) of violent death among the previous personalities of the twin cases, but it was not significantly different from that (51%)
of a much larger series of other cases.

In 34 of the 42 cases we were able to learn whether the previous personalities had died at the same or different times. In 62% of the cases for which we had
this information, they had died at the same time or at least on the same occasion,
such as in a vehicular accident. In the remaining 38% of cases, the previous personalities had died at different times, sometimes at widely separated intervals,
even many years apart.

We tried to learn whether a subject who remembered a previous relationship
with his or her co-twin in which the previous personality remembered by the subject had been dominant would show dominance over the co-twin. We did not find
it easy to obtain sufficiently reliable information on the feature of dominance,
especially because some of the twins were still young when we studied their
cases, and there had been little time or opportunity for either twin to express any
tendency to dominate the co-twin. Nevertheless, among 11 cases for which we

obtained satisfactory information on this feature, we found that a dominant twin remembered the life of a dominant previous personality in every instance.

The most important points of the analysis of these twin cases are the high incidence of a personal relationship between the previous personalities of a twin pair and the high incidence of a personal relationship between the previous personalities and the twins' parents. (I remind readers again of the heavy loading of our series of twin cases with instances in Burma.) Next I will present summaries of three more cases of twins, two from Sri Lanka and one from Burma.

Sivanthie and Sheromie Hettiaratchi were born in Galle, Sri Lanka, on November 3, 1978. Their parents were Amarapala Hettiaratchi and his wife, Yasawathie. They lived in the village of Pitadeniya, which is 14 kilometers north of Galle.

Sivanthie was the older twin by 5 minutes. She was born with a prominent birthmark on her abdomen. It was an area of heavily increased pigmentation. When she was about 4 years old, it measured about 2 centimeters in length and 1 centimeter in width at its widest extent (*). Sheromie had no birthmark. From analysis of the twins' blood groups and subgroups we learned that they were fraternal (dizygotic) twins.

Sivanthie was the first of the twins to speak about a previous life. At the age of about 2½ she began referring to another home where she said that she had a father, mother, and younger sister. She made many statements about the previous life, including descriptions of how in the previous life she had been shot while jumping into the sea. When she spoke about being shot, she pointed to the birthmark on her abdomen. She asked to go to "my home" and also spoke about a temple at a place called Yatigala, which is close to Galle and about 15 kilometers from Pitadeniya. When Sivanthie was about 3½, Yasawathie took her to the temple at Yatigala. There Sivanthie made some further statements about the previous life she was remembering. Also at about this time she said that in the previous life her name had been Robert.

Sivanthie talked about a previous life for about a year during which Sheromie said nothing. Sivanthie's statement that she had been called Robert, together with her description of being shot as Robert and jumping into the sea, identified the person she was talking about as a well-known insurgent called Robert, who had been killed by the police during the insurgency in Sri Lanka of April 1971. Robert had had a close friend called Johnny. Word of what Sivanthie had been saying spread to Robert's family (who lived near Galle) and from them to the family of Johnny. One of Johnny's younger brothers, Gnananadasa, then went to Pitadeniya to see the twins. When Sheromie saw him, she said: "My younger brother has come." Then she too began to talk about a previous life, that of Johnny. Thereafter, the twins often talked about the lives of Robert and Johnny. Although Sivanthie had not earlier identified Sheromie as Johnny reborn, at least to the knowledge of adults in the family, once Sheromie had begun to talk about the life of Johnny, each twin fully recognized the other as from the previous lives.

After Gnananadasa's visit to the twins, they subsequently met other members of both Johnny's and Robert's families. The twins recognized some of these persons correctly. Sivanthie, unaided according to Godwin Samararatne, who was with her, showed the way along a tortuous path (which I later traversed myself) to the place where Robert had tried to escape from the police, the details of which I will mention later.

The families of Robert and Johnny fully accepted the twins as being these men reborn. No member of their families—and we interviewed 12 in all—expressed any doubts concerning the twins' claims.

Before describing the twins' unusual behaviors, I will describe the lives and deaths of Johnny and Robert. Johnny, like Robert, had been an insurgent; he was in fact the leader of the insurgents in the Galle area. He and Robert were best friends and well known in the area to be homosexuals. They were not, however, effeminate. They engaged skillfully in such activities as swimming and climbing trees (an essential skill in the harvesting of coconuts).

Robert had no steady work, but did odd jobs here and there, repairing houses or working as a mason. Johnny became employed at a factory for making spectacle frames. Amarapala Hettiaratchi was employed at the same factory, and be became acquainted with Johnny there. He invited Johnny, and Robert also, to attend his wedding.

Robert and Johnny belonged to the underemployed segment of Sri Lankan youth from which members of the 1971 insurgency movement were largely recruited. The insurgents succeeded in concealing their intentions and preparations so well that when they struck—mainly at police stations in the hope of obtaining more arms—the government was to some extent taken by surprise. It reacted swiftly, and within a few weeks the insurgency had been suppressed—brutally and with excessive force, it was generally thought afterward. Robert and Johnny had at first hidden themselves, but then for some reason decided to move away from Galle. Someone tipped the police, who arrested them at the bus station in Galle.

They were taken to the police station and interrogated. Robert had the idea that he might escape by jumping into the sea. He offered to show the police where the insurgents had hidden bombs on a hill, which had a cliff with the sea directly beneath it. The police accepted his proposal. Informants saw Robert with his hands handcuffed behind his back being led to this hill by a group of policemen. A short time afterward, a shot was heard, and the policemen returned without Robert. The police officers later said that Robert had kicked one of them, tried to butt another with his head, and was going to jump into the sea and escape. (This was not necessarily a foolish plan, because Robert was an excellent swimmer and might have survived even with his hands restrained.) One of the policemen then shot him, and his body fell or was pushed into the sea.

The police were so angry over Robert's almost successful attempt to deceive them that, back in the police station, they beat up Johnny until he died. They then hanged his body by the feet and subsequently cremated it. Many of the details I have mentioned—and others—figure in the statements that Sivanthie and Sheromie made.

I have already explained that the twins' father, Amarapala, had known Johnny well and had had some acquaintance with Robert. The circumstances of the deaths of Robert and Johnny were also well known in the community. It is therefore unlikely that Sivanthie and Sheromie made any statements about matters outside their parents' normal knowledge. This is not to say that they obtained their knowledge of the lives and deaths of Robert and Johnny from their parents or from any other normal source. The insurgency had occurred about 10 years before Sivanthie began to talk about a previous life, and I think it improbable that she heard references to it that would account for her detailed knowledge of the life of Robert.

The twins' unusual behavior forms as important a part of their case as their statements. They showed several markedly masculine traits. They liked to wear T-shirts and to roll them up above the waist so that their abdomens and lower chests were exposed; Robert and Johnny had sometimes rolled up their T-shirts as the twins did. They sometimes wore pieces of cloth that they would arrange like a man's sarong. They also urinated standing up, as boys do, until their mother checked this. They both liked to climb trees and play with bicycles, generally considered masculine activities; however, they also played with dolls and sometimes at cooking.

In addition to the types of play I have already mentioned, the twins also played at making bombs with clay. When asked of what bombs were made, they mentioned some of the ingredients that would have gone into the crude bombs that the insurgents had made.

The twins also sometimes showed "adult attitudes." They put sticks in their mouths and pretended to be smoking cigarettes. (Robert and Johnny had smoked cigarettes.) They both said they had beards and sometimes stroked their faces as if feeling a beard's growth.

Both of the twins had a noticeable phobia of loud noises, of persons wearing khaki (which the police usually wore in Sri Lanka), and of Jeeps, a vehicle commonly driven by the police and army there.

In addition to the prominent birthmark on Sivanthie, the twins showed differences of complexion and physique that corresponded to similar differences between Robert and Johnny. Sheromie was noticeably darker in complexion than Sivanthie (*); Johnny had been darker than Robert. Robert was shorter and stockier than Johnny; and Sivanthie was shorter and stockier than Sheromie (*).

Indika and Kakshappa Ishwara were born on October 24, 1972, at Weligama, Sri Lanka. Their parents were M. D. Ishwara and his wife, Swarnawathie. They lived in a village about 7 kilometers from Weligama. Indika was born 5 minutes before Kakshappa. I later determined, from analyses of their blood groups and sub-groups, that they were identical (monozygotic) twins. About a year after the twins' birth Indika was found to have a nasal polyp, which to some extent obstructed the airway on the left side of his nose (*). Kakshappa had no nasal polyp.

When the twins were about 3 years old, they began to speak about previous lives. Kakshappa spoke first and said that he had been shot by the police. He made a few other statements that suggested the life of an insurgent. For example, he mentioned a place, Elpitiya, that was known to have been a center of the insurgency movement of 1971 (which I mentioned in connection with the cases of the Hettiaratchi twins). For a reason I have never understood, the twins' family laughed at Kakshappa, and he never spoke again about a previous life. His case remains unsolved.

Indika, on the other hand, had much to say about the life that he remembered. He gave many details including names of people and places, and these made it comparatively easy to verify his statements. He said that he had lived in a place called Balapitiya and had attended school in (the nearby town of) Ambalangoda. Other details that Indika mentioned suggested that he was talking about the life of a young schoolboy.

Weligama is on the south coast of Sri Lanka, about halfway between Galle and the city of Matara. Balapitiya and Ambalangoda are on the western coast of the island, 6 kilometers apart. Ambalangoda is about 45 kilometers from Weligama "as the crow flies," but farther by road or rail. M. D. Ishwara had a friend in Weligama who worked in Ambalangoda, and this man, with the details stated by Indika, easily found a family of Balapitiya whose oldest (and then only) son, Dharshana, had died in Colombo after a short illness, on January 24, 1968. He was not quite 11 years old.

Dharshana's father, R. L. Samarasekera, learned about Indika's statements and went to Weligama to meet him. He quickly became convinced that Indika had detailed knowledge about the life of Dharshana Samarasekera. Subsequently, R. L. Samarasekera made two further visits to Indika at Weligama. On the second visit, he brought three other members of the family with him, and Indika recognized them. Indika also visited the Samarasekeras at Balapitiya.

Indika was credited with 36 statements about the previous life, all, so far as I could learn, made before the two families had met. Of these 36 statements, 31 were correct, 1 was unverified, 2 were incorrect, and 2 were doubtful. Some of the statements were applicable to many families in Sri Lanka, but others were much more specific, such as Indika's mention of an older sister called Malkanthie and a person he called "Aunt Chilies." The last person indicated had cooked chilies for Dharshana, who was her nephew. Indika did not state Dharshana's name, at least initially. He did, however, say that in the previous life he had been called "Baby Mahattaya," which translates best as "little master." This had been Dharshana's pet name.

Some of Indika's doubtful and incorrect statements were "near misses." For example, he said that he had a bicycle, which was wrong. Dharshana, however, had a tricycle, and he sometimes used his father's bicycle; in a childlike way

Dharshana might have come to think of this bicycle as his own. Another example occurred in Indika's statement that the family had a calf. They owned no calf, but other persons brought their calves to graze on the extensive grounds in the Samarasekeras' compound.

Indika's most surprising statement referred to an event that even Dharshana's family knew nothing about. During his second visit to the Samarasekeras' house in Balapitiya, Indika was noticed to be going around another house in the same compound as if looking for something on the wall of a concrete drain. Finally, he found what he was looking for and pointed to the name *Dharshana* and the date *1965*, which had been scratched into the concrete while it was still soft. Dharshana, who did this, had told no one in the family what he had done, and none of them had noticed Dharshana's name in the concrete until Indika showed it to them.

Our investigation of this case began within a few weeks of its development. We reached the scene of the case just a little too late to make a written record of Indika's statements before they were verified, yet soon enough so that the informants were remembering events that had happened recently. I am convinced that the two families had had no prior acquaintance before the case developed. I say this not only because of the considerable geographical distance separating them, but because they belonged to widely different social strata. Indika's family were rural persons; his father was a shopkeeper who could not speak English. In contrast, Dharshana's father was a government employee who spoke English. Apart from these circumstances, Dharshana had been a young schoolboy, virtually unknown outside his family, friends, and school. His death at such a young age was saddening, but included nothing sensational that might have carried news of it to Weligama.

I come now to the important differences in the behavior of Indika and Kakshappa. There were nine of these. Indika was religious, but Kakshappa was indifferent to religion. Indika was calm and gentle in manner; Kakshappa tended to be tough and inclined even to be violent. Indika expected to be addressed respectfully, but Kakshappa was indifferent about how he was addressed. Indika was more intelligent than Kakshappa and had an excellent memory, better than Kakshappa's. Indika liked schoolwork and was good at it; Kakshappa was indifferent to schoolwork and weak at studies. Indika sometimes talked to himself; Kakshappa did not do this. Indika had a phobia for vehicles, but Kakshappa did not. Indika was inclined to be somewhat aloof from other members of the family; Kakshappa was affectionate toward other members of the family. Indika was more fond of chilies than Kakshappa.

Several of these differences require some explanatory comment. Indika's expectation of being addressed respectfully corresponded to Dharshana's status as the oldest son (and during his life the only son) in the family. Indika's aloofness from his family may have derived from his memories of the special status he remembered Dharshana to have had in his family. He probably made matters worse by openly saying that his "Ambalangoda mother and father" (as he called

R. L. Samarasekera and his wife) gave him more affection than his parents. (I do not think this was true, but he thought it was and said so.) As for Indika's phobia of vehicles, this may have derived from Dharshana's having observed, about a month before he died, a child run over and killed by a truck. It could also have been related to the fact that when Dharshana became ill, he was transported in vehicles to hospitals, first in Galle and then in Colombo, where he died.

Although they had the marked differences that I have described, the twins got along well together. They were closer to each other than to their older brothers. They sometimes quarreled, but if anyone else then intervened, they resisted such an intrusion into their affairs. As the twins became older, some of the differences between them that I have described diminished or disappeared.

As I mentioned, Dharshana had died after a brief illness. His death certificate attributed his death to "viral encephalitis" and "cardiorespiratory failure." The records at the Colombo General Hospital, where he had died, had been destroyed after 10 years. It happened, however, that R. L. Samarasekera had preserved a piece of paper on which the doctor who had treated Dharshana in Galle had scribbled some notes about the treatment given at Galle. The notes included the words: "Nasal feed 6 hourly given." This shows that Dharshana had been fed through a nasal tube at Galle (and perhaps at Colombo also). I believe that Indika's nasal polyp may correspond to the irritation produced by the nasal tube in Dharshana's nose.

Although they were one-egg twins, Indika and Kakshappa did not look alike; their faces were quite different (*). Indika's face did not resemble Dharshana's, as I could observe in a photograph of him that R. L. Samarasekera made available to us (*).

Maung Aung Ko Thein and Maung Aung Cho Thein were born in Moulmein, Burma, on July 5, 1970. Their parents were U Hla Thein and Daw Khin Kyi. Maung Aung Ko Thein made only two statements about a previous life, and Maung Aung Cho Thein made none. They were identified as being the reincarnations of two persons known to their mother. This conclusion was based on two dreams she had had, as well as on differences in the twins' physical appearances and behaviors.

Maung Aung Cho Thein was identified as the reincarnation of Daw Hla May, a relative of Daw Khin Kyi. She had been a prosperous owner and manager of a family mill. She was Chinese. During her final illness, Daw Khin Kyi had moved in with Daw Hla May and had nursed her until she died.

Maung Aung Ko Thein was identified as the reincarnation of an Indian paddy farmer, Sunder Ram, who had brought his paddy to Daw Hla May's mill to be milled. He had also sometimes worked with his cart on hire for other persons. Maung Aung Ko Thein's two statements referred to Sunder Ram's activity as a farmer and a carter.

Maung Aung Ko Thein had a birthmark, a small area of increased pigmentation on the upper part of the helix of one ear (*). This corresponded to a hole pierced for an earring and was similar to the birthmarks on Maung Nyunt (Chapter 24) and Edward Taylor (Chapter 8). In addition, Maung Aung Ko Thein had markedly darker skin than that of Maung Aung Cho Thein (*). The differences in complexion corresponded to the differences in complexion between Chinese and Indian people. The former are usually light-complexioned, the latter nearly always more heavily pigmented.

The twins showed markedly different behaviors in a number of respects. Of these the most important was the tendency of Maung Aung Cho Thein to act in a superior, dominating manner toward his brother. For his part, Maung Aung Ko Thein seemed to accept unquestioningly his brother's attitude of superiority. Their behaviors accorded with those of the well-to-do mill owner and the poor paddy farmer who had brought his rice to her mill.

I return now to the case of Gillian and Jennifer Pollock. As I mentioned in Chapter 23, they were identical (monozygotic) twins. As do most such twins, they had nearly identical facial appearances when they were young, although in later life they were more easily distinguishable.

Jacqueline, whose life Jennifer remembered, had had a flat mole (nevus) on her left flank, and Jennifer had a similar one at the same location. Neither Joanna nor Gillian had a mole at that location.

When Jacqueline was about 3 years old, she fell, and her face hit a bucket that wounded her on the forehead, above her right eye. The wound required three stitches, and a scar remained. I saw a photograph of her that clearly showed this scar (*). Jennifer was born with a birthmark at the site of the scar on Jacqueline's forehead. A photograph taken at the twins' baptism shows this birthmark (*). It persisted into Jennifer's adulthood (*). Gillian had no birthmark on her forehead. Neither Gillian nor Jennifer had any birthmark that might have derived from the injuries that had killed Joanna and Jacqueline.

26

GENERAL DISCUSSION

Having said earlier in Chapter 15 all that I have to say about the authenticity of the cases and the reasons I have for favoring reincarnation as the best interpretation of the stronger ones, I will add nothing further on these topics here. In this final chapter I will address some of the implications of reincarnation and discuss some of the processes that may be involved, if it occurs.

The concept of reincarnation seems otiose to persons, including many scientists, who believe that present knowledge of genetics and the influence of the uterine and postnatal environments adequately explain, or will eventually explain, all aspects of human personality. I cannot advance the merits of reincarnation as a contributory factor in the composition of human personality by exposing the limitations of genetics and environmental influences, but a brief review of these limitations may make some readers more receptive than they would otherwise be to additional explanatory factors—such as reincarnation.

Genes provide the instructions for the production of proteins or, more accurately, for the ingredients of proteins. If they fail to code for an essential protein or if they instruct for one that is abnormal, a clear-cut genetic disease may result. Examples of these effects are sickle cell disease, hemophilia, and Marfan syndrome. Such diseases are called monogenic, and they comprise a small proportion of all diseases. Geneticists describe other diseases or physical features that have a genetic component as polygenic, meaning that several or many genes must contribute to the condition. (Stature is a typical example of a condition said to be polygenic.) As I pointed out in Chapter 17, however, even diseases that seem most obviously genetic, such as Marfan syndrome, show a wide variation in the manifestations of the disorder, not only between members of different affected families, but between the different members of one affected family. To account for these variations geneticists have introduced the concept of "modifier genes," but (as I mentioned earlier) these are for the most part imagined, not specified. Their use evokes memories of the epicycles introduced into Ptolemaic cosmology to account for otherwise inexplicable anomalies in astronomical observations.

I said earlier that genes provide the instructions for proteins. From them alone, however, we have no understanding of how proteins develop their complicated three-dimensional structure. Even less does our knowledge of genes explain how proteins and other metabolites become organized into cells and then into highly differentiated tissues and the complicated organs that comprise our bodies. Present knowledge of genes tells us almost nothing about embryology and morphology, which is the science of the forms that organisms have. Some geneticists are not modest in assuring us that they will in due course supply all the information we need to understand embryology and morphology. This amounts to a promissory note with no immediate cash value, and in the meantime we are free to consider the possibility of other contributory factors.

Geneticists have allied themselves with other biologists who believe that natural selection provides a sufficient explanation of evolution. This neo-Darwinian synthesis now has hegemonic power among biologists. In recent decades a noticeable minority of biologists have drawn attention to the insufficiencies of neo-Darwinism. Defenders of current biological orthodoxy have tried to stigmatize these dissidents as detractors of Charles Darwin. Such pejorative labeling does not, however, answer the objections of the critics of neo-Darwinism; and surely we deduct nothing from the achievement of Darwin by saying that his theory explains much but not all that we need to understand about evolution.

As for the influence of the environment, it has long been held by nearly all psychologists and psychiatrists that infancy and early childhood are times of special plasticity in the formation of a human personality. Events of that period, it is believed, may permanently influence and thus make or mar the personality for life. This belief has a long history. In modern times it was the single belief on which psychoanalysts and behaviorists could agree; both accepted it as axiomatic. Where, however, is the evidence for such an unshakeable conviction? There is none, although there does exist a considerable body of published, if neglected data that show the reversibility of the effects of seemingly damaging events of early childhood. I do not deny that earlier events leave traces that may influence later ones. What I deny is that human personality is more vulnerable in infancy and childhood to the effect of injurious events than it is in later phases of life.

Having drawn attention to the limitation of genetics and environmental influences in early life, I need now to state that I do not propose reincarnation as replacing these factors. I regard it as a third factor that may fill some of the gaps in the knowledge we presently have about human personality and, as the cases of this work suggest, about the human body also. I turn now to some of the implications of the acceptance of reincarnation as such a contributing factor.

The most important consequence would be acknowledgment of the duality of mind and body. We cannot imagine reincarnation without the corollary belief that minds are associated with bodies during our familiar life, but are also independent of bodies to the extent of being fully separable from them and surviving the death of their associated body. (At some later time, they become associated with a new physical body.) In saying this I declare myself an adherent of interactionist dualism. This concept has an ancient history, but in recent times perhaps derives most from ideas of William James and Henri Bergson. They suggested that the brain acts as a filter between stimuli reaching it and consciousness, which needs only a limited amount of information. Proponents of dualism do not deny the usefulness of brains for our everyday living; but they do deny that minds are nothing but the subjective experiences of brain activity. How minds and brains interact during life is part of the agenda for future research; but that is equally true of the claims confidently made by many neuroscientists who assert that minds are reducible to brain activity. We need not, however, be misled into mistaking claims for accomplishments.

If dualism be accepted, we must consider where minds would exist between terrestrial lives. I believe that we are obliged to imagine a mental space that, necessarily, differs from the physical space with which we are ordinarily familiar. I think that introspection can show that our thoughts occupy a mental space distinguishable from physical space, even while we are alive; but I will not review the evidence for that here. What I can say here, however, is that a mental space where discarnate personalities might exist between terrestrial lives is not only conceivable, but has already been conceived and described in considerable detail by several philosophers familiar with the evidence of the phenomena now called paranormal.

This space or realm where discarnate personalities might sojourn between lives would be markedly different from that with which we, while living, are familiar. Not having there the aid of our present sensory equipment, our perceptions in that realm would differ greatly from those to which we are accustomed. We should not be without thoughts, however, and indeed mental images might abound. Existence there might have features that would seem familiar to persons who have given more than average attention to their dreams, to persons who have taken such drugs as mescaline and LSD, and to some persons who have come close to death and survived.

If we accept the possibility that a personality can survive physical death and reincarnate, we may ask what features might be transmitted from one life to another. I have found it helpful to use the word *diathanatic* (which means "carried through death") as a term for subsuming the parts of a deceased person that may reach expression in a new incarnation. So what parts would be diathanatic? The cases I have described tell us that these would include: some cognitive information about events of the previous life; a variety of likes, dislikes, and other attitudes; and, in some cases, residues of physical injuries or other markings of the previous body.

The information conveyed, or at least expressed, by the child is much reduced from that of the previous personality. Despite wide variation among the subjects, on the whole they express little of all that must have been in the mind of the person whose life they remember. As I mentioned in Chapter 1, more than a few children, although identified with a particular previous personality through dreams or birthmarks, say nothing whatever in words about their presumed previous life.

The unusual behavior seemingly carried over from the previous life is also comparatively attenuated. This is equally true of the physical phenomena. The baby with birthmarks or birth defects is not born (there seem to be a few exceptions) with the open wounds from which the previous personality died; the baby's body shows marks or defects at the sites of these wounds, but not the wounds themselves (except for occasional minor bleeding or oozing of fluid).

We may understand better the loss through death of some or much of the previous personality by using the distinction between *personality* and *individuality*. By individuality I mean all the characteristics, whether concealed or expressed, that a person might have from a previous life, or previous lives, as well as from this one. By personality I mean the aspects of individuality that are currently expressed or capable of expression. For example, if I had learned to speak Swahili in a previous life, but had no opportunity or ability to speak it in this one, an aptitude to do so would form part of my individuality, but would not be part of my personality. If I were to try to learn Swahili in this life, however, the experience of my previous life might make it easier for me to learn the language than it would otherwise be.

I will next consider three ways in which experiences of a previous life might influence the physical body of a new incarnation. Selection of one's parents, when feasible, would be one method. In the cases of William George, Jr., Corliss Chotkin, Jr., and Wijeratne, the previous personalities predicted that they would be reborn to certain parents; and children of the selected parents gave evidence of remembering the lives of these persons. In addition, we have seen in many cases that a previous personality had strong ties of affection to the subject's parents. Our studies of twins especially show this, but many other cases do so also. Bonds of affection may have acted, therefore, to bring a previous personality to rebirth in a particular family, even when no one formally predicted this. The evidence for this makes the cases of the children who remember previous lives parallel in this respect to those of telepathy between living persons. These occur much more frequently between persons having an affectionate relationship than they do between strangers.

A discarnate personality might also influence its next physical body by somehow screening and selecting fertilized ova (zygotes or conceptuses) or embryos. Apart from any other relevant feature, such selection seems to be essential if the personality is not to change sex from one life to another. Even in Burma where 26% of cases are of the sex-change type, some selection of the right physical body would be essential in most cases. I am unable to state how a discarnate personality would achieve this purpose. I may mention, however, the possibility— which has some supporting evidence—that psychological factors may modify the vaginal secretions of a woman to give more or less advantage to Y chromosome-carrying sperms (from which males derive) compared with X chromosome-carrying ones. If a discarnate personality can—as some cases suggest—induce unusual cravings in pregnant women, perhaps it can also influence the physical body of a mother-to-be so as to favor or disfavor conceptuses of one or the other sex.

With the two methods of influencing the body of the next incarnation that I have just described—selection of parents and selection of conceptuses or embryos—the reincarnating personality has to accept whatever body its new parents can provide. The third method of influence that I am supposing includes a direct effect of the discarnate personality on the new body. It is the one that the cases of this work mainly suggest. I mean effects on the embryo or fetus that to some extent reproduce the physical attributes of the last physical body. I am referring to birthmarks, birth defects, and some of the other physical features of the subject that correspond to similar ones of the previous personality. Any such direct influence implies some kind of template that imprints the embryo or fetus with "memories" of the wounds, marks, or other features of the previous physical body. The template must have a vehicle that carries the memories of the physical body and also the cognitive and behavioral ones. I have suggested the word *psychophore* (which means "mind-carrying") for this intermediate vehicle. (I know that many religions that include a belief in reincarnation have words to describe such an intermediate vehicle; I have thought it helpful, however, to coin a new word that would avoid linking our still rudimentary scientific study of reincarnation to any religion.)

The existence between terrestrial lives is therefore, according to this view, a corporeal one, but the psychophore would not be made of the material substances with which we are familiar. I cannot say of what it would be made. To suggest that it would be made of some nonmaterial mind stuff adds little information, but I cannot propose anything more specific.

I mentioned earlier that birthmarks and birth defects are not exact reproductions of bleeding wounds; they might be considered mental scars of such wounds that affect another physical body. The reproductions, however, often lack exactitude. The new body may show an influence from the previous body that exceeds the area involved in the previous body's wounds. One example of this occurred in the case of Lekh Pal Jatav (Chapter 17). Hukum Singh, whose life Lekh Pal remembered, had all the fingers of his right hand severed, but not its thumb; yet Lekh Pal's right thumb was just as much involved in the birth defect of his right hand as were his other fingers. Another example of an effect larger in area than that of the original lesion occurred in the case of Selma Kılıç. The previous personality in her case died of nephritis, and Selma also had nephritis. In addition, however, Selma had a large birthmark on her back at the level of a kidney, suggesting an influence from the disease of kidneys in the previous life much more extensive than the area of Selma's kidneys. These and other cases suggest to me that the psychophore has the properties of a field or, more probably, a collection of fields that carry the physical and other memories of the previous life and more or less reproduce them by acting on the embryo or fetus of the new body. The English scientist Michael Faraday first introduced the concept of a field in physics to assist in understanding the relationship between magnetism and electricity; schoolchildren become familiar with fields when they observe how iron filings organize themselves around the poles of a magnet. In the early 1920s several European biologists used the concept of a field to help in understanding the successive development from a fertilized ovum of first an embryo, then a fetus, and finally a baby. Morphogenetic fields have been imagined as governing the development of the forms that organs and the whole body of which they are the parts will have. The cases whose subjects have birthmarks and birth defects suggest that discarnate personalities may sometimes influence the morphogenetic fields and modify a physical body toward some correspondence with that of a previous life.

Readers may reasonably ask whether there exists any evidence for a vehicle such as the psychophore apart from the cases of children who remember previous lives and who have birthmarks or birth defects. The answer is not much. Nevertheless, certain cases of apparitions furnish some relevant evidence. Most apparitions appear fleetingly, and the perception lasts only a few seconds; there is no interaction between the percipient and the perceived figure. Such cases have value, but not as evidence of a corporeal entity; they may derive from telepathy between the percipient and a living person, the latter (usually called an agent) being often in some extremely stressful situation, perhaps on the edge of death. There is, however, a small number of cases in which an apparitional figure stays longer where it is seen and reacts appropriately to the person or persons who see it, perhaps moving from one person to another with seeming purposefulness. Sometimes the appearing figure remains long enough so that it can be seen from different angles and even walked around. It is difficult to explain such cases as these without supposing that the appearing figure is present and somehow incorporated. We cannot say how it is incorporated, except that it must be in some nonmaterial substance.

Some additional evidence for a vehicle that I have called a psychophore comes from the occurrence of phantom limbs in congenital amputees—persons born with parts of limbs missing. Until the last few decades such phantom limbs were thought to be rare—and by some authors impossible. Nevertheless, among 101 congenital amputees studied in the 1960s, 18 had phantoms.

Some readers may think I should cite here as evidence of a psychophore the frequent experiences of persons who come close to death and survive and who say afterward that while they were apparently unconscious and near death they moved away from their physical body and seemed to be in a nonmaterial body, one that could perceive other (living) persons, even though these persons could not perceive the experient in his or her new location. Therein lies the difficulty. So long as the experience provides no feature that someone else—some person other than the principal subject—can report, we have no objective evidence of a nonmaterial vehicle. The perceived body seemingly detached from the physical one may be only a subjective mental image.

Apparitional cases that the investigators of these experiences call "reciprocal cases" may provide such objective evidence. In such cases—reports of which are regrettably rare—the primary percipient reports later that he or she traveled to another place and saw and perhaps spoke to a person there, usually a loved relative or close friend. The person he or she claims to have visited later reports having seen the primary experient (and perhaps spoken to him or her) at the time the primary percipient had the experience.

Acceptance of reincarnation as the best explanation for the cases releases a mass of questions about processes for which we have as yet no answers. A hint toward one factor comes from the high incidence of violent death among the previous personalities in the cases. A violent death is nearly always sudden and unexpected; it is premature, because even an old person killed violently would have lived longer if he or she had not been so killed; and it is nearly always accompanied by physical suffering. An analysis that we made suggests the importance of these features. We sometimes learned (or could estimate) the interval between a fatal wound and the previous personality's death. Among the 62 cases for which we had the necessary information, the interval between the two events was less than 5 minutes in 36 (58%), and less than 24 hours in another 17 (27%). These two groups thus together accounted for 85% of the cases. It seems, therefore that a fatal wounding shortly before death may have a facilitating influence in the occurrence of birthmarks and birth defects that correspond to wounds in a previous life.

This leads to the question of how violence acts as a facilitator. I believe that it does this by concentrating attention on the affected part of the body. In Chapter 2 I emphasized the importance of intense concentration in the occurrence of stigmata, and I believe this is also important in maternal impressions. A person suddenly shot, stabbed, or struck will inevitably concentrate attention on the wounded part. (This may not happen immediately; I know there are cases of wounded soldiers and athletes continuing their activities for some time after being wounded.)

Increased attention to a part of the body may also figure importantly in birthmarks not related to wounds inflicted violently. I can suppose, for example, that Dominic Nwachi (the presumed previous personality in the case of Augustine Nwachi) thought much as he was dying about the swollen, gangrenous toes that were causing his death. Another example of concentrated attention occurs in the cases with birthmarks corresponding to holes pierced for earrings. The piercing is nearly always conducted with some ceremony; often it is a rite of passage that focuses the child's attention on the pierced holes, as do also the earrings that are thereafter worn in the holes.

I do not clearly see an influence from increased attention in experimental birthmarks and birth defects. The person marked or mutilated is on the verge of dying or actually dead when the body is marked or cut. We presume such a person incapable of attending to anything. A few subjects have claimed to have observed their body after dying, and one might suppose in these cases that they gave special attention to any mark or cut made on the body. That is, after all, what the person making the mark or mutilation expects, and it may be that all dying persons give concentrated attention to their dead bodies, but only a few can later remember this.

A further question arises about the morphological correspondence between the mental images conveyed in the psychophore and the parts of the new body that it influences. We have to suppose a close anatomical collocation of the two, not too different from that between a hand and a glove that fits it. Mental images held with concentration may, as I have suggested, intensify the influence of the psychophore, but the latter may also convey to the new body abnormalities in the previous personality's body of which he or she could have had no conscious mental image. Gunshot and other wounds to the head from behind could not be seen by a victim before he or she died; nor could wounds on the back. Such wounds could not form part of visually originated mental images. The physical body itself may therefore be able to imprint such abnormalities on the psychophore without passage through a stage of conscious mental imagery.

I have now said the little that I can say at present about processes whereby birthmarks and birth defects corresponding to wounds and other marks on a previous personality occur. It remains for me to conclude by reiterating both some of my disclaimers and some of my conclusions.

Among disclaimers I wish most to emphasize that in presenting the cases of this book I am not presuming to offer an explanation for *all* birthmarks and birth defects. I dare hope that the cause I favor for the cases I have described, which is that they derive from previous lives, may have a wider applicability and throw light on other instances of birthmarks and birth defects; but this is a matter to be decided by further research, not by assertion from me. I also repeat that I do not propose reincarnation as a substitute for present or future knowledge of genetics and environmental influences. I think of it as a third factor contributing to the formation of human personality and of some physical features and abnormalities. I am, however, convinced that it deserves attention for the additional explanatory value that it has for numerous unsolved problems of psychology and medicine.

Until now I have said nothing about the potential value of the idea of reincarnation in reducing the fear of death that is so prevalent in the West. It has been wisely said that the question of a life after death is the most important one that a scientist—or anyone—can ask. I have deliberately kept this aspect of reincarnation in the background until now, because I am well aware that the fear of death may encourage a belief in a life after death. It is true that many of us want to believe in a life after death, but our wish that something may be true does not make it false. We may, after all, be engaged in a dual evolution—of our bodies and of our minds or souls.

SOURCES OF
ADDITIONAL
INFORMATION

A. The monograph of which this is a synopsis is *Reincarnation and Biology: A Contribution to the Etiology of Birthmarks and Birth Defects*. Westport, CT: Praeger Publishers, 1997.

B. Case Reports of the 19th Century and Early Decades of the 20th Century

1897   Hearn, Lafcadio. The rebirth of Katsugoro. In *Gleanings in Buddha-fields: Studies of hand and soul in the Far East*. Boston: Houghton Mifflin.

1898   Fielding Hall, H. *The soul of a people*. London: Macmillan.

1924   Sunderlal, R. B. S. Cas apparents de réminiscences de vies antérieures. *Revue métapsychique* no. 4, pp.302-07.

c. 1927 Sahay, K. K. N. *Reincarnation: Verified cases of re-birth after death*. Bareilly: N. L. Gupta.

C. Books and Related Articles with Case Reports (often detailed) by Ian Stevenson

1960a   The evidence for survival from claimed memories of former incarnations. Part I. Review of the data. *Journal of the American Society for Psychical Research* 54:51-71.

1960b   The evidence for survival from claimed memories of former incarnations. Part II. Analysis of the data and suggestions for further investigations. *Journal of the American Society for Psychical Research* 54:95-117.

1966   Cultural patterns in cases suggestive of reincarnation among the Tlingit Indians of Southeastern Alaska. *Journal of the American Society for Psychical Research* 60:229-43.

1970   *Telepathic impressions.* Charlottesville: University Press of Virginia. (Also published in 1970 as vol. 29 of the *Proceedings of the American Society for Psychical Research.*)

1974   *Twenty cases suggestive of reincarnation.* 2d rev. ed. Charlottesville: University Press of Virginia. (First published in 1966 as vol. 26 of the *Proceedings of the American Society for Psychical Research.*)

1975   *Cases of the reincarnation type. Vol. 1, Ten cases in India.* Charlottesville: University Press of Virginia.

1975   The belief and cases related to reincarnation among the Haida. *Journal of Anthropological Research* 31:364-75. (Reprinted with revisions in *Journal of the American Society for Psychical Research* 71:177-89, 1977.)

1977   *Cases of the reincarnation type. Vol. 2, Ten cases in Sri Lanka.* Charlottesville: University Press of Virginia.

1977   The explanatory value of the idea of reincarnation. *Journal of Nervous and Mental Disease* 164:305-26.

1980   *Cases of the reincarnation type. Vol. 3, Twelve cases in Lebanon and Turkey.* Charlottesville: University Press of Virginia.

1983   *Cases of the reincarnation type. Vol. 4, Twelve cases in Thailand and Burma.* Charlottesville: University Press of Virginia.

1985   The belief in reincarnation among the Igbo of Nigeria. *Journal of Asian and African Studies* 20:13-30.

1986   Characteristics of cases of the reincarnation type among the Igbo of Nigeria. *Journal of Asian and African Studies* 21:204-16.

1987   *Children who remember previous lives.* Charlottesville: University Press of Virginia.

1988a   Three new cases of the reincarnation type in Sri Lanka with written records made before verification (with Godwin Samararatne). *Journal of Nervous and Mental Disease* 176:741.

1988b   Three new cases of the reincarnation type in Sri Lanka with written records made before verification (with Godwin Samararatne). *Journal of Scientific Exploration* 2:217-38. (A more detailed report of the cases reported in 1988a.)

1989   A case of the possession type in India with evidence of paranormal knowledge (with Satwant Pasricha and Nicholas McClean-Rice). *Journal of Scientific Exploration* 3:81-101.

1989   A case of severe birth defects possibly due to cursing. *Journal of Scientific Exploration* 3:201-12.

1990   Phobias in children who claim to remember previous lives. *Journal of Scientific Exploration* 4:243-54.

1992   A new look at maternal impressions: An analysis of 50 published cases and reports of two recent examples. *Journal of Scientific Exploration* 6:353-73.

1993   Birthmarks and birth defects corresponding to wounds on deceased persons. *Journal of Scientific Exploration*. 7:403-10.

D. Publications by Other Scientists Who Have Independently Investigated the Cases of Children Who Remember Previous Lives

1988   Mills, Antonia. A preliminary investigation of reincarnation among the Beaver and Gitksan Indians. *Anthropologica* 30:23-59.

1988   Mills, Antonia. A comparison of Wet'suwet'en cases of the reincarnation type with Gitksan and Beaver. *Journal of Anthropological Research* 44:385-415.

1989   Mills, Antonia. A replication study: Three cases of children in northern India who are said to remember a previous life. *Journal of Scientific Exploration* 3:133-84.

1990a   Mills, Antonia. Moslem cases of the reincarnation type in northern India: A test of the hypothesis of imposed identification. Part I: Analysis of 26 cases. *Journal of Scientific Exploration* 4:171-88.

1990b   Mills, Antonia. Moslem cases of the reincarnation type in northern India: A test of the hypothesis of imposed identification. Part II: Reports of three cases. *Journal of Scientific Exploration* 4:189-202.

1990   Pasricha, Satwant. *Claims of reincarnation: An empirical study of cases in India*. New Delhi: Harman Publishing House.

1991   Haraldsson, Erlendur. Children claiming past-life memories: Four cases in Sri Lanka. *Journal of Scientific Exploration* 5:233-61.

1991   Keil, Jürgen. New cases in Burma, Thailand, and Turkey: A limited field study replication of some aspects of Ian Stevenson's research. *Journal of Scientific Exploration* 5:27-59.

1994   Mills, Antonia. "Rebirth and identity: Three Gitksan cases of pierced-ear birthmarks." Chap. 13 in *Amerindian rebirth: Reincarnation belief among North American Indians and Inuit*, edited by A. Mills and R. Slobodin, pp. 211-41. Toronto: University of Toronto Press.

1994   Mills, Antonia; Haraldsson, Erlendur; and Keil, Jürgen. Replication studies of cases suggestive of reincarnation by three independent investigators. *Journal of the American Society for Psychical Research* 88:207-19.

1995   Haraldsson, Erlendur. Personality and abilities of children claiming previous-life memories. *Journal of Nervous and Mental Disease* 183:445-51.

1996   Keil, Jürgen. Cases of the reincarnation type: An evaluation of some indirect evidence with examples of "silent" cases. *Journal of Scientific Exploration* 10:467-85.

INDEX

This index is one of subjects (topics) and also of cases, which are indicated by the *first* names of the subjects. Other persons, such as investigators, are listed with surnames first. The names of subjects of cases of the reincarnation type are given in italics, other names in roman type. Burmese subjects are listed without honorifics, although these are used in the text.

The following abbreviations have been used:

CORT   Case (or cases) of the reincarnation type
PL   Previous life
PP   Previous personality
S   Subject (of a case)

IAN STEVENSON is Carlson Professor of Psychiatry and Director of the Division of Personality Studies at the Health Sciences Center, University of Virginia. He has published nine books on his research since 1966, two of which have been translated into French, German, and Japanese.

ISBN 0-275-95188-X

90000>

EAN

9 780275 951887

HARDCOVER BAR CODE